OTC MEDICATIONS

Symptoms and Treatments of Common Illnesses

Second Edition

A. LI WAN PO

BPharm, PhD, FRPharmS
FPSNI, FRSC, FRSS
The School of Pharmacy
University of Nottingham

and

G.LI WAN PO

MB, CHB
General Practitioner, Lincoln

**Blackwell
Science**

© A. Li Wan Po and G. Li Wan Po, 1992, 1997

Blackwell Science Ltd
Editorial Offices:
Osney Mead, Oxford OX2 0EL
25 John Street, London WC1N 2BL
23 Ainslie Place, Edinburgh EH3 6AJ
350 Main Street, Malden
  MA 02148 5018, USA
54 University Street, Carlton
  Victoria 3053, Australia

Other Editorial Offices:

Blackwell Wissenschafts-Verlag GmbH
Kurfürstendamm 57
10707 Berlin, Germany

Blackwell Science KK
MG Kodenmacho Building
7–10 Kodenmacho Nihombashi
Chuo-ku, Tokyo 104, Japan

First edition published 1992
Reprinted with updates 1993
Second Edition published 1997

Set in 10/13pt Ehrhardt
by DP Photosetting, Aylesbury, Bucks
Printed and bound in Great Britain by
Hartnolls Ltd, Bodmin, Cornwall

The Blackwell Science logo is a trade mark of Blackwell
Science Ltd, registered at the United Kingdom Trade
Marks Registry

DISTRIBUTORS

Marston Book Services Ltd
PO Box 269
Abingdon
Oxon OX14 4YN
(*Orders:* Tel: 01235 465500
       Fax: 01235 465555)

USA
Blackwell Science, Inc.
Commerce Place
350 Main Street
Malden, MA 02148 5018
(*Orders:* Tel: 800 759 6102
           617 388 8250
       Fax: 617 388 8255)

Canada
Copp Clark Professional
200 Adelaide Street West, 3rd Floor
Toronto, Ontario M5H 1W7
(*Orders:* Tel: 416 597 1616
           800 815 9417
       Fax: 416 597 1617)

Australia
Blackwell Science Pty Ltd
54 University Street
Carlton, Victoria 3053
(*Orders:* Tel: 03 9347 0300
       Fax: 03 9347 5001)

A catalogue record for this title is available
from the British Library

ISBN 0-632-04046-7

Library of Congress
Cataloging-in-Publication Data
is available

Tables from *Dietary Reference Values for Food Energy and Nutrients for the United Kingdom*, HMSO Press, are
reproduced with the permission of the Controller of HMSO.

Contents

Preface to the first edition

Health professionals are often required to provide answers to patients' questions about a variety of health matters. However, often the same busy professionals find it difficult to have access to the necessary information to ensure that the advice given is rational. This book is written in an attempt to meet some of their information needs with respect to self-limiting conditions and some remedies available for their symptomatic relief. As such, this book can be regarded as a sequel to *Non-Prescription Drugs* by the same authors (ALWP).

Since publication of *Non-Prescription Drugs*, a number of major developments have occurred in this field. In particular, a number of countries, including the United Kingdom, have introduced a limited prescription list. Simultaneously, a number of prescription drugs have been delisted to become non-prescription drugs within specific formulations and dose ranges. Notable examples are ibuprofen, hydrocortisone, terfenadine, loperamide, clotrimazole and miconazole. Additionally, with the institution of a more rigorous regulatory review of product licences, manufacturers have sponsored a large number of pharmacological and clinical projects to provide the necessary data for supporting their applications for new product licences. The resulting body of new information has made the writing of this book both more interesting and more laborious.

The answers given in the text are based on the authors' distillation of the current literature. In providing short answers to questions, simplifications are often necessary. Inevitably also, with time, new information will reduce the validity of some of the answers given and it is the authors' hope that the book will reawaken the reader's interest in the primary literature.

In compiling this book we have attempted to make it easy to use. Therefore we have used an alphabetical entry which runs along the top corner of each page. This entry includes both product categories (e.g. analgesics and vitamins) and disease categories (e.g. migraine and diarrhoea). A more detailed index is included at the end of the book.

Within each section we have included a subsection on *Precautions and when to refer* and one on *Product options*. We hope that readers will find these useful as quick references to potentially serious problems and to products which are worthy of consideration for particular ailments. In identifying first-choice products we have taken into account current expert opinion but the final list is necessarily subjective. Monocomponent products are preferred to polycomponent ones unless there is clear evidence of additive or synergistic effects. In some product categories, such as antifungal agents, the choice is clear. In others there is no such obvious choice. For example, with common cold products, the ideal product is very much based on many other factors such as concurrent medication and disease. For these product groups we have made no recommendations. In yet other categories of products, such as those containing vasoconstrictor agents, no choice is made because in our view none of those listed are safe and/or effective.

A more detailed discussion of non-prescription products is given in the book *Non-Prescription Drugs* by the same publishers.

The authors will welcome comments from readers relating to both the format and contents of this book. Additional questions or topics for inclusion in any subsequent editions of the book will also be warmly received.

Preface to the second edition

A number of prescription only drugs have been down-regulated to pharmacy only status recently. Moreover since publication of the last edition of this book, numerous important studies on the evaluation of over the counter drugs have appeared in the literature. It was therefore felt inappropriate by both our publishers and ourselves to reprint the first edition without a thorough revision; hence this second edition. This has taken longer than we anticipated and we are sorry that there has been a discontinuity in the availability of the book. Indeed, at several points during the revision, we thought of drawing a line, only to be defeated by the introduction of yet more new OTC drugs. Such is the current speed of developments in this area.

The rapid developments are a result of consumers asking to have more control over their own therapies and governments recognising that making more effective remedies available for self-medication can substantially reduce the burden placed on national health services or insurance health schemes through better use of existing health-care networks such as that represented by community pharmacists.

We hope that the summaries we have provided are as evidence-based as possible. While there is an increasing amount of novel information being generated about the drugs which are considered in this book, knowledge about the efficacy of many existing therapies is still sparse. The necessary randomized, controlled studies have yet to be undertaken. In our evaluations, we have accepted this. As long as the risks are likely to be insignificant, we have adopted a permissive position and have not been too critical of the use of well accepted but unproven remedies. We have nonetheless indicated at the appropriate places, which therapies are validated and which are not whenever possible. This position recognises the importance of both evidence-based practice and the contribution which placebo effects can make to the efficacy of pharmacotherapies particularly in the context of self-medication.

A number of readers have been kind enough to feed us back some comments on the first edition of this book and we hope that the revisions which we have made reflect the importance which we attach to their observations. Further comments are invited.

Introduction: prescribing OTC medications

General advice about prescribing non-prescription drugs

(1) Prescribe only when necessary and when benefits are likely to outweigh the risks.

(2) Be particularly careful when recommending non-prescription drugs to pregnant women, infants and the elderly (see below).

(3) Watch out for potential drug–drug interactions and remember to take into account prescribed medication.

(4) Remember that some drugs may be excreted in breast milk in sufficient amounts to cause distress in the nursling.

(5) When recommending proprietary or branded medication ensure that the patient is not receiving the same drug under a different name, particularly with analgesics and sympathomimetic agents.

(6) When in doubt refer.

(7) Discourage chronic use of non-prescription medication (laxatives, nasal decongestants and cough mixtures).

(8) Watch out for drug abuse (laxatives, cough mixtures, opiate-containing anti-diarrhoeal mixtures and hyoscine-containing products such as travel-sickness tablets).

Prescribing OTC products for the elderly

(1) Avoid anticholinergics in the elderly (hyoscine, some antihistamines).

(2) Check concurrent medication particularly carefully (monoamine oxidase inhibitors, antihypertensives, anticoagulants, cytotoxics).

(3) Avoid constipating drugs (aluminium-containing antacids, opiates).

(4) Take care when recommending CNS depressants (e.g. some antihistamines).

(5) Avoid formulations with high sodium content (antacids, effervescent tablets).

(6) The elderly are particularly susceptible to the gastro-intestinal side-effects of non-steroidal anti-inflammatory drugs.

Prescribing OTC products during pregnancy

(1) Do not give iodine-containing products (antibacterial lozenges, iodine antiseptics, some cough mixtures).

(2) Avoid large doses of caffeine (tonics, analgesics).

(3) Do not give aspirin.

(4) Avoid theophylline (cold products).

(5) Do not give ibuprofen

(6) Avoid excessive doses of vitamin A.

(7) Take care with codeine preparations.

(8) Avoid excessive use of topical anti-parasitic formulations (scabicides, pediculicides).

(9) Avoid piperazine.

(10) Avoid unnecessary drugs, particularly during the first trimester.

Prescribing OTC products during breast feeding

(1) Do not give iodine-containing products (some antibacterial lozenges, iodine antiseptics, some cough mixtures).

(2) Avoid large doses of caffeine (tonics, combination analgesics).

(3) Avoid ephedrine-containing formulations (decongestants).

(4) Do not give aspirin..

(5) Avoid large doses of theophylline-containing cold products.

(6) Avoid phenolphthalein-containing products (laxatives).

Prescribing OTC products for children

(1) Avoid use of oral and nasal decongestants.

(2) Avoid use of antispasmodics.

(3) Avoid use of antihistamines as sedatives.

(4) Avoid use of antidiarrhoeals other than rehydration fluids in children.

(5) Do not give aspirin to children.

(6) Avoid formulations containing sugar.

(7) Avoid prophylactic use of antiparasitic formulations (scabicides, pediculicides).

Medicines recently down-regulated

Drug Year	Therapeutic category/ indication	Non-prescription products
Acrivastine (1993)	Antihistamine H_1	
Acyclovir (1993)	Anti-viral agent; cold sores	Zovirax Cold Sore Cream
Aluminium chloride hexahydrate (1994)	Antiperspirant	Anhydrol Forte, Driclor
Alverine citrate (1996)	Irritable bowel syndrome	Relaxyl
Astemizole (1988)	Antihistamine H_1	Hismanal, Pollon-eze
Beclomethasone dipropionate (1994)	Corticosteroid	Beconase Hayfever
Carbenoxolone granules		
Carexomer iodine (1995)	Disinfectant	Iodosorb powder

Drug Year	Therapeutic category/ indication	Non-prescription products
Cetirizine (1993)	Antihistamine H_1	Zirtek
Cimetidine (1994)	Antihistamine H_2	Tagamet 100 Tagamet Dual Action
Cromoglycate sodium (cromolyn sodium) eye drops (1994)	Hay-fever	Opticrom Allergy, Brol-eze
Dextranomer topical (1987)	Disinfectant (wound care)	Debrisan
Dextromethorphan controlled release oral form (1989)	Antitussive	
Diclofenac diethylammonium	Topical analgesic	Voltarol Emulgel
Dihydrocodeine/paracetamol combination (1992)	Analgesic	Paramol
Econazole vaginal (1992)	Vaginal candidiasis	Gyno-pevaryl
Famotidine (1994)	Antihistamine H_2	Pepcid AC
Felbinac Gel (1996)	NSAID	Traxam Gel
Fluconazole (oral) (1995)	Anti-candidal agent (vaginal candidiasis)	Diflucan One
Flunisolide nasal spray (1994)	Corticosteroid (Hay-fever)	Syntaris Hayfever
Hydrocortisone 1% topical (1987)	Corticosteroid	Dermacort, Lanacort, Hc45
Hydrocortisone topical dermal (1994)	Extension of indications to atopic eczema	
Hydrocortisone anal and rectal (1994)	Extension of product range to haemorrhoidal products	Anusol Plus HC Proctofoam HC
Hydrocortisone (1994) 2.5% buccal pellets	Mouth ulcers	Corlan pellets
Hydrocortisone/crotamiton (1994)	Combination antipruritic	Eurax HC
Hydroxyzine (1995)	Antihistamine H_1	
Hyoscine butylbromide (1992)		Buscopan
Ibuprofen (1983)	Analgesic; non-steroidal	Nurofen, Proflex, Ibugel
Ibuprofen gel (1988)	NSAID	Ibuleve
Ibuprofen sustained release (1988)	NSAID; analgesic	Proflex SR
Isoconazole (1992)	Vaginal candidiasis	
Isosorbide dinitrate (1988)	Anti-anginal	Cedocard 20

Drug Year	Therapeutic category/ indication	Non-prescription products
Ketoconazole 2% shampoo (1995)	Anti-dandruff shampoo	Nizoral
Ketoprofen gel (1993)	NSAID	Oruvail gel
Loperamide (1983)	Anti-diarrhoeal agent	Arret, Imodium, Diocalm Ultra
Loratadine (1992)	Antihistamine H_1	Clarityn
Mebendazole (1989)	Antivermifuge	Ovex
Miconazole vaginal (1992)	Vaginal candidiasis	Femeron
Minoxidil 2% topical (1994)	Alopecia	Regaine
Nizatidine (1996)	Antihistamine H_2	Axid AP
Oxethazine (1994)	Surface anaesthetic in antacid formulation	Mucaine
Piroxicam gel (1994)	NSAID	Feldene P Gel
Pyrantel Embonate (1995)	Anti-vermifuge	Combantrin
Ranitidine (1994)	Antihistamine H_2	Zantac 75
Terfenadine (1983)	Antihistamine H_1	Triludan
Tioconazole vaginal (1994)	Vaginal candidiasis	
Triamcinolone 0.1% oral paste (1994)	Mouth ulcers	Adcortyl in Orabase S

Counter-prescribing protocols

Alertness is required whenever the prescription of a medication is being considered. In a busy environment, it is easy to overlook what in hind-sight are obvious warning signs or elements of good prescribing practice. For this reason prescribing protocols are often recommended, and indeed organizations such as the Royal Pharmaceutical Society of Great Britain expect protocols to be used in day-to-day counter-prescribing. ENCORE is a mnemonic for a general protocol to be used when responding to symptoms; it was developed specifically in response to criticisms of poor standards of counter-prescribing made by the Consumer's Association. The essential steps are summarized by the letters of the mnemonic as follows:

Explore   the nature of the symptom; other associated symptoms; con-
                 current medication; possibility of serious disease; ascertain
                 identity of patient.

No medication   remember that this is an option. Indeed in some cases a medi-
                 cation is contra-indicated.

Care   be particularly careful when dealing with certain groups of

	patients, notably the very young, the elderly and pregnant and lactating mothers.
Observe	be alert; look for tell-tale signs; a very ill-looking patient may need to be referred.
Refer	potentially serious cases; persistent symptoms; patients at increased risk of complications.
Explain	patients are more likely to take advice, if appropriate explanation is provided.

Acne

Who suffers most from acne?

Acne is essentially a disease of the teenager and the young adult. Acne typically starts at the onset of puberty and its severity usually declines sharply beyond the teenage years. Most acne cases are under control by the time the patients reach 30 years of age. There is no evidence to show that one sex is any more susceptible to acne than the other.

How common is acne?

Acne is one of the commonest dermatological problems. Surveys have shown that this disorder affects about 75% of teenagers and adults below 30. It has been estimated that about a third of all patient visits to dermatologists are for this condition.

What causes acne?

The current view is that acne is a multifactorial disease. The following theories have been put forward.

Hormonal imbalance

The temporal association of the development of acne with puberty suggests a hormonal involvement. However the levels of the sex hormones or their relative ratios in acne patients and in acne-free patients do not show any consistent difference and current theory suggests that the sebaceous glands (Figure 1) may be more responsive to androgenic hormones in acne patients than in control subjects.

Microbial colonisation of sebaceous follicles

Some supporting evidence for this theory is provided by the effectiveness of antimicrobial agents in acne. However, a number of studies using both surface and pilosebaceous sampling of bacteria have produced little evidence for an increased microbial colonisation of the skin or its appendages in acne patients. There is also no evidence to show that the skin flora is changed in acne. The micro-organisms of the sebaceous follicle appear to be limited to the same four genera (*Propiono-bacterium, Staphylococcus, Micrococcus and Pityrosporum*) irrespective of whether acne is present or not. The attention of most of the microbiologists active in the study of acne has been mainly on the gram positive non-motile rod *Propiono-*

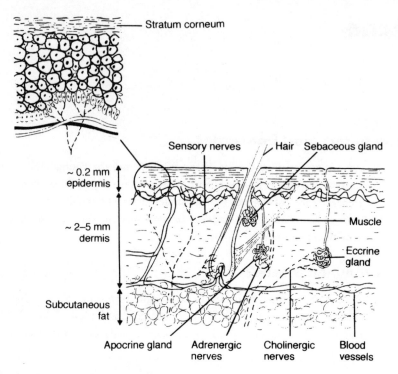

Fig. 1   The skin and its appendages.

bacterium acnes which was previously described as *Corynebacterium acnes* type I. *Cor. acnes* type IIa and type IIb are now known as *P. avidum and P. granulosum* respectively. It is possible that current methods for microbiological typing and culture are not sensitive and/or selective enough to identify organisms which may be involved in acne.

Inflammatory response to micro-organisms or to their metabolic products

P. acnes is known to have the potential to initiate inflammatory responses when injected into keratinous cysts. The mechanisms put forward to explain this include immunostimulation by cell wall mucopeptides, complement activation and chemotaxis by its metabolic products. One intriguing observation against this theory is that only a small proportion of follicles develop into acne even in severe cases.

Formation of abnormally cohesive sebum

The presence of cohesive plugs are readily seen as comedoes (whiteheads and blackheads) in acne patients. Why such plugs are formed is not understood.

Irritation by breakdown products of sebum

In acne, the skin is often greasy and it has been suggested that breakdown products of sebum irritate the skin and initiate or intensify acne. There is indeed some evidence to show that antibiotic treatment often reduces the proportion of free fatty acids in serum concurrently with an improvement in acne. However, the fact that not all subjects with greasy skins and the same degree of bacterial colonization of the skin develop acne, indicates that the theory cannot stand alone. Studies with lipase inhibitors have shown that although the levels of free fatty acids can be reduced with these agents, the severity of acne is not improved.

Treatment options

Products available for the treatment of acne contain agents which can be classified according to their modes of action as shown in Table 1. It can be seen that some agents act by more than one mechanism. In addition to chemically active agents some formulations also include abrasives (polyester, silica, aluminium oxide) for the physical loosening of the keratin plugs and surfactants for the removal of excess sebum.

Table 1 Mode of action of active ingredients commonly included in topical anti-acne formulations.

Drug	Main modes of action
Allantoin	Keratolytic (?)
Benzalkonium chloride	Antimicrobial
Benzoyl peroxide	Keratolytic Antimocrobial
Cetylpyridinium chloride	Antimicrobial
Cetyltrimethyl ammonium bromide (Cetrimide)	Antimicrobial
Chlorhexidine	Antimicrobial
Ethyl lactate	Antimicrobial (indirect)
Miconazole	Antimicrobial
Nicotinamide	Anti-inflammatory
Octaphonium chloride	Antimicrobial
Phenol	Antimicrobial
Potassium hydroxyquinoline sulphate	Antimicrobial
Retinoic acid (all trans)	Keratolytic Stimulates cell turnover
Salicylic acid	Keratolytic
Triclosan	Antimicrobial
Vibenoid	Keratolytic

Recently, nicotinamide gel has been introduced for the treatment of acne. Does it work and what is its mechanism of action?

Nicotinamide was evaluated as a potential anti-acne compound because of its structural similarities with retinoic acid, which (in its various isomeric forms) is known to be effective in acne. While there is some suggestion that the product is effective, the published data are insufficient to enable a rigorous assessment of its efficacy relative to other commonly used anti-acne remedies, most notably benzoyl peroxide. Until more clinical data is made available, nicotinamide gel must be regarded as a second-line treatment.

How can acne scars be avoided?

When a case of acne is considered, an important principle to note is that vigorous treatment is required whenever there is severe inflammation and whenever there are large cysts, nodules and pustules. These would suggest involvement of the deeper dermal tissues and potentially irreversible damage and scar formation. Non-prescription remedies will need to be supplemented with oral antibiotics and in the severest and most recalcitrant of cases, with retinoids.

Can acne scars be chemically removed?

Some recent claims have been made that topically applied retinoids may reverse some of the scars seen in acne. These claims have yet to be validated.

Does the menstrual cycle affect the severity of acne?

Cyclic flare-ups are indeed commonly seen in female acne sufferers. Typically, the worsening appears 7–10 days before menstruation. Mid-cycle flares are also seen in some patients. The premenstrual worsening is generally ascribed to increased concentrations of progesterone during the luteal phase of the cycle. Why progesterone which is not androgenic should be acnegenic is not understood.

Do certain drugs induce acne?

Androgenically active drugs clearly have the potential to stimulate acne. Anabolic agents and some contraceptive agents fall into this category. Iodides, lithium and anticonvulsant compounds are widely regarded as potentially acnegenic but the evidence is generally poor and a recent study in fact showed that the anticonvulsant compounds did not cause or exacerbate acne.

Do certain foods induce or exacerbate acne?

Again the evidence is poor. Items such as chocolates which are widely held as being acnegenic have in fact been shown not to be so in a controlled trial. Some patients will insist that certain specific foods definitely cause a worsening of their acne and it is difficult to refute their claims as self-induced stress may well exacerbate acne, possibly through depression of the immune system.

Precautions and when to refer

(R) Patients should be referred if inflammation is severe and/or cysts are present.

(R) Acne in the very young and in non-teenage patients presenting with acne for the first time.

(R) Acne flare-ups in patients receiving ACTH, phenobarbitone, isoniazid and iodides.

(!) Keratolytic agents (Table 1) may cause an apparent worsening of the acne before improvement is observed.

Product options

Benzoyl peroxide-containing products:
Acetoxyl gel	Acnecide gel	Acnegel
Benoxyl Cream and Lotion	Boots Mediclear Cream	Panoxyl Aquagel and Gel

Benzoyl peroxide combination products (second-line):
Acnidazil Cream	Quinoderm Cream and Lotion

Allergy

What is allergy?

Allergy refers to any abnormal reaction or hypersensitivity to substances to which one is exposed. Well-known examples include allergy to pollen (hay-fever), allergy to cosmetic agents and allergy to nickel. In medical science, allergy usually refers to conditions in which an antigen and a specific biochemical immune response can be identified. Thus conditions such as sun-allergy and lactose intolerance, commonly described as allergies by the wider public are not considered to be true allergies by immunologists.

What causes allergy?

True allergies are caused by substances (antigens) which the body recognises as being foreign. Upon such molecular recognition by lymphocytes and antibodies, an inflammatory process and further production of antibodies are initiated by the activated lymphocytes. In conjunction with non-antigen specific cells, such as the phagocytes, and molecules from the complement system, the lymphocytes and antibodies cooperate to eliminate the antigens. In normal circumstances these functions take place without significant disturbance as the immune system regulates itself to trigger a response appropriate for the antigenic load encountered. In allergies, the control exerted by the immune system breaks down and abnormal reactions are initiated. In hay-fever for example, excessive rhinorhoea, itch and inflammation of the conjunctival and nasal tissues are observed.

Is there any cure for allergies?

Allergies do resolve spontaneously. For example, hay-fever invariably gets better as the patient grows older so that very few elderly patients suffer from hay-fever. In some cases, the allergy is more persistent (e.g. nickel allergy) and continuous avoidance of exposure to the allergen is necessary. In most allergies, treatment is aimed at suppressing the disturbing symptoms.

Are there useful non-prescription drugs for allergies?

Effective non-prescription remedies are available for the symptomatic relief of certain allergies (e.g. hay-fever and insect stings) but not for others (e.g. nickel allergy and the more serious allergies such as allergic asthma). However, even in the latter cases, symptomatic treatment by non-specific remedies, such as emollients in nickel allergy, may be helpful. Generally, although topical antihistamines are theoretically useful for alleviating allergic itch, they are not recommended as they may themselves induce hypersensitivity reactions.

Further references

See entries for antihistamines, hay-fever and eczema.

Anaesthetics (topical)

Are anaesthetic agents useful for topical analgesia?

Local anaesthetics such as lignocaine and benzocaine produce analgesia when applied to mucous membranes and to broken skin. They are only slowly effective when applied to intact skin, often requiring over 1 hour occlusion before any perceptible effects. Therefore, except for specific applications such as preoperative treatment for skin grafting, local anaesthetics are not useful for application to skin areas covered with stratum corneum. They are, however, highly effective for relieving pain or itch affecting areas covered with mucous membranes. Pain or itch in the buccal cavity or in the genito-labial areas can therefore be conveniently treated with local anaesthetics. For those areas, other standard topical agents such as the salicylates, nicotinates and capsaicin would be unsuitable as they are too irritant.

How do local anaesthetics work?

Local anaesthetics exert pain relief by reversibly blocking the action potential in nerves. This is achieved by preventing the increase in sodium permeability, arising from the painful stimulus, probably through blockade of the sodium channels. Use of different stereoisomers of the local anaesthetics suggests the presence of two sites of binding on the sodium channel. One lignocaine isomer, for example, produces a much stronger dose-dependent block than the other.

Which is the best topical anaesthetic to use?

Benzocaine and lignocaine are the best-established local anaesthetics for topical use and would therefore be safest, although a wide range of compounds are available (Table 2). Some may be preferable to benzocaine and lignocaine for specific purposes, although strict comparisons to take into account length and duration of

Table 2   Types of anaesthetic agents used topically.

Esters	Amides
Amethocaine	Bupivacaine
Benzocaine	Dibucaine (Cinchocaine)
Procaine	Etidocaine
Tetracaine	Mepivacaine
	Prilocaine

action have yet to be conducted. Most of the comparative work has been on speed of onset of activity.

Product options

Xylocaine 4% Topical Solution
Xylocaine Antiseptic Gel

Xylocaine Gel
Xylocaine Spray

Analgesics (oral)

What causes pain?

Pain may be caused by a whole variety of toxic stimuli. Three types of pain fibres are known, depending on whether they respond to pressure (mechano-pain receptors), temperature (thermo-pain receptors) or chemicals (chemo-pain receptors). Chemo-pain receptors are most often involved in commonly encountered pain. As a result of tissue damage, a number of chemical mediators, including bradykinin, histamine, prostaglandins, 5-hydroxytryptamine and proteolytic enzymes, are released. These chemical agents may damage the nerve endings and sensitise or stimulate them to produce pain. Prostaglandins, in particular, sensitise nerve receptors to the other algogens.

The chemical mediators released may also decrease the sensitivity threshold of the mechanosensitive and thermosensitive pain receptors so that normally painless pressure or temperatures become unbearable. Ischaemia is known to induce pain, probably also through a chemical pathway such as accumulation of lactic acid. Muscle spasm may cause pain by inducing ischaemia and hence also lactic acid accumulation. Signals arising from the interactions between the chemicals, pressure or temperature with the pain receptors are then conveyed to the central nervous system to be processed as pain.

What is referred pain?

Pain is often felt at a site remote from the tissues causing the pain. Such pain is known as referred pain. The explanation for referred pain is that pain fibres from the viscera synapse in the spinal cord with some of the same neurons which receive dermal pain fibres. Therefore pain arising from the viscera is confused by the integrating centre as being pain originating from the skin.

Treatment options

Aspirin, benorylate, ibuprofen and paracetamol are available as single-agent non-prescription analgesic products in the United Kingdom. Codeine and caffeine are secondary agents commonly included in compound analgesic formulations. Salicylamide, sodium salicylate and lithium sulphate are now rarely used as analgesics.

How do the oral analgesics work?

The oral analgesics do not all share the same mode of action. Codeine is a narcotic analgesic with its site of analgesic action in the central nervous system. Sensitivity of the pain receptors and nerve conduction do not seem to be affected. Aspirin and ibuprofen produce pain relief by interfering with prostaglandin formation from arachidonic acid. Those two analgesics probably also exert their antipyretic activity through the same mechanism in the brain.

Paracetamol has now overtaken aspirin as the most widely used mild analgesic agent. Despite this, there is still little known about its precise mechanism of action. While there is growing support for the view that paracetamol exerts its activity mainly by central mechanisms, the basis for the central activity is unsatisfactorily explained. The central analgesic effect appears to be independent of endogenous opiods and one popular view is that paracetamol selectively inhibits cyclo-oxygenase in the central nervous system but not in the periphery. This selectivity of action may account for the drug's effectiveness as an antipyretic agent as well as for its lack of activity as an anti-inflammatory agent.

While paracetamol interferes with nerve conduction, experiments using animal tissues show that this effect is only seen at concentrations well above doses equivalent to those used in clinical practice. Paracetamol, however, is known to block impulse generation at bradykinin-sensitive chemoreceptors which evoke pain. Based on current evidence the conclusion must therefore be that both peripheral and central mechanisms are involved in the analgesic activity of paracetamol.

Benorylate, being an aspirin and paracetamol prodrug, shares the same mode of action as the latter two drugs.

Is the prophylactic use of paracetamol against fever after immunization justified?

While some doctors and nurses advise that this should be done, most authorities are of the view that prophylactic use of paracetamol is not justified. However, should fever and painful swelling develop after immunizations then treatment with appropriate doses of paracetamol is rational.

Are codeine-containing combination analgesic products worthwhile?

Codeine is a centrally-acting analgesic while aspirin, paracetamol and ibuprofen are all peripherally-acting analgesic products. Therefore a combination of codeine with one of the peripheral analgesics is logical. The available evidence, however, suggests that codeine is not a very effective analgesic at non-prescription doses. However, compound codeine or analgesic formulations may perform better than paracetamol or ibuprofen on its own. The improvement in efficacy may be largely due to an enhanced placebo effect although a modest effect over and above the latter is also possible. One recent meta-analysis suggested that while this may be so, the improvement is not clinically significant even at codeine doses several times higher than those found in OTC products.

Does caffeine enhance the performance of analgesic tablets?

Clinical trials carried out to evaluate the comparative performance of analgesic tablets, with and without caffeine, have yielded conflicting results. A recent review of the literature on the subject considered 30 clinical studies meeting generally accepted criteria of a randomized, unbiased, controlled clinical trial. By pooling the data, the authors concluded that the overall pooled relative potency estimate of caffeine-containing products relative to caffeine-free controls, was 1.41, with 95% confidence limits of 1.23–1.63. The suggestion was that in order to obtain the same degree of pain relief from an analgesic without caffeine, a dose approximately 40% higher than one with caffeine would be required. However more recent meta-analyses suggest that this may not be clinically meaningful.

Should analgesic-caffeine combinations then be preferred to the simpler formulations?

There is little justification for using analgesic-caffeine combination products as first-line analgesics although a case can be made for their occasional use when a simple analgesic is claimed to have been tried without success. The German Prescription Committee was sufficiently concerned by reports of abuse that it considered banning all combination analgesics from non-prescription use. It is claimed that abusers are taking caffeine-containing products as 'pick-me-ups' without taking adequate account of the large doses of analgesics consumed at the same time. No such controls appear to be envisaged by the Committee on Safety of Medicines since abuse of combination products is less of a problem in the UK.

Are there any useful herbal analgesic products?

Willowbark contains salicylic acid and for this reason is included in many herbal analgesic products. It is doubtful, however, whether the small doses present in standard products are of any therapeutic value. Salicylate-sensitive patients should, however, avoid such products. An interesting herb of potential analgesic value is feverfew. Some laboratory data suggest that it has anti-prostaglandin activity as well as anti-platelet activity not related to its anti-prostaglandin effects. Current interest centres on its use in migraine. While there is some data to show that it may be useful in migraine, further good clinical data is required. Other herbal remedies (e.g. passion fruit) with claimed analgesic activities are probably no more than mere placebos. For self-limiting pain, placebos are surprisingly active.

Does aspirin cause Reye's syndrome?

Reye's syndrome is a rare acute encephalopathy which is commonly fatal. The condition typically occurs after viral infections such as influenza and chickenpox. In survivors, neurological damage may be permanent. One of the earliest reports suggesting an association between the condition and aspirin intake dates back to 1965. Since then the association has been consistently reaffirmed by a number of different studies. Despite methodological problems and the fact that association does not necessarily mean causation, the drug regulatory authorities in a number of countries, including the USA and the UK, are sufficiently convinced to recommend restrictions in the sale of aspirin. In the UK aspirin usage is now essentially confined to the adult population. Since such restrictions of use, the incidence of Reye's syndrome in children has decreased significantly. Benorylate, which is metabolized to aspirin, should also be avoided by children.

Do non-steroidal anti-inflammatory drugs interfere with the action of antihypertensive drugs?

There is now sufficient data to show that non-steroidal anti-inflammatory agents interfere with the action of antihypertensive drugs. Indomethacin and piroxicam have been implicated but other non-steroidal anti-inflammatory drugs such as sulindac and aspirin appear to be safe. The position of ibuprofen is less clear because of contradictory evidence and until this is resolved it seems prudent to avoid ibuprofen in patients receiving antihypertensive drugs. Paracetamol is a suitable alternative for those patients.

Are analgesics safe in pregnancy?

All drugs should be avoided, if at all possible, during pregnancy. However, epidemiological data suggest that paracetamol is most probably safe in pregnancy. One recent study, however, suggests that it may enhance the teratogenic effect of phenytoin. Aspirin has been associated with perinatal problems and on theoretical grounds aspirin, benorylate and ibuprofen, because of their anti-prostaglandin activities, may cause premature closing of the ductus arteriosus.

Is it true that non-steroidal analgesic drugs may cause weight gain?

A recent study investigating the effect of ibuprofen on blood pressure control by propranolol and bendrofluazide indicated that ibuprofen may cause weight gain in some individuals but the interaction with the antihypertensive drugs used is unclear. The acute weight gain was, however, not associated with any changes in blood pressure.

Which analgesics should asthmatics avoid?

Aspirin and ibuprofen are both known to cause bronchoconstriction in some patients and asthmatic patients are a well-known at-risk group to this adverse reaction and several deaths have been reported. There appears to be cross-reactivity between aspirin, ibuprofen and the other non-steroidal anti-inflammatory agents, suggesting that the mechanism may be linked with inhibition of arachidonic acid metabolism in the lung. Cross-sensitivity with tartrazine has also been reported. Paracetamol appears to be a safer analgesic for the asthmatic, although idiosyncratic reactions have occasionally been reported too. A number of respiratory physicians are now of the view that while caution is justified, ibuprofen is not necessarily contra-indicated in asthmatic patients unless they are hypersensitive to aspirin or NSAIDs.

What is the placebo effect?

The placebo effect is a highly complex phenomenon describing relief of symptoms induced by chemical entities or procedures which theoretically have no inherent pharmacological activities. Examples of the placebo effect include relief of common cold symptoms by normal saline, relief of headache by lactose tablets and relief of abdominal pain by diagnostic procedures. Some conditions and indeed most symptoms, for which non-prescription remedies are recommended, are subject to high placebo effects. Analgesic branding, for example, has been shown to have an effect on the effectiveness of analgesics in relieving pain.

How does acupuncture provide pain relief?

Much research has been carried out on acupuncture and although it is now generally accepted that the technique can provide pain relief for a variety of clinical problems, the precise mechanisms involved are still unclear. The involvement of humoral factors is supported by cross-circulation experiments in animals as well as by reversal of the analgesia by naloxone, an opiod receptor-blocking drug. Electro-acupuncture has also been shown to lead to the release of met-enkephalin and ß-endorphin into the cerebro spinal fluid. Changes in 5-hydroxytryptamine levels in the central nervous system may also be involved. The involvement of the neural pathways is demonstrated by the abolition of acupuncture analgesia by injection of local anaesthetics at the site of needle insertion or acupoints.

Precautions and when to refer

(!) Potential drug-drug interactions

Aspirin	Anticoagulants	Increased risk of bleeding
	Phenytoin	Enhanced effect
	Sodium valproate	Enhanced effect
	Methotrexate	Increased toxicity
	Spironolactone	Antagonism of diuretic effect
	Acetazolamide	Reduced excretion and increased risk of toxicity

	Probenecid	Effect reduced
	Sulphinpyrazone	Effect reduced
	Lithium	Reduced excretion
Benorylate	As with aspirin although less pronounced	
Ibuprofen	Lithium	Reduced excretion
	Antihypertensive agents	Antagonism of effect and increased risk of renal problems
	Diuretics	Increased risk of renal problems
Paracetamol	Glucose test	

(!) Potential drug-disease interactions

Aspirin	Not to be used in children under 12
	Avoid in patients with history of gastrintestinal ulceration
	Avoid in gout and haemophilia
	Avoid during breast feeding (Reye's syndrome)
	Care with asthmatics
	Care in the presence of renal problems
	Care with diabetics as aspirin exerts a small hypoglycaemic effect
Benorylate	As with aspirin and paracetamol
Ibuprofen	Care in the presence of renal problems
	Avoid during pregnancy
	Avoid in aspirin-sensitive patients

(!) General recommendations

Aspirin, ibuprofen and paracetamol are first-line general analgesic products. The equivalent doses are 600 mg, 400 mg and 100 mg respectively.

Children should not be given aspirin because of its association with Reye's Syndrome.

Patients hypersensitive to aspirin should avoid it as well as ibuprofen.

Combinations of aspirin and paracetamol are no better than the single agents on their own.

Codeine may enhance the analgesic efficacy of paracetamol, aspirin and ibuprofen but, at OTC doses, this effect is negligible.

Dihydrocodeine does not produce any clinically meaningful improvement in the analgesic effects of paracetamol.

Caffeine is not an effective analgesic adjuvant.

Buffered formulations should be restricted to occasional single-day use.

Antihistamines such as doxylamine and diphenhydramine add little to analgesic formulations and may cause drowsiness.

Oral aspirin and ibuprofen formulations should be avoided in those with a history of gastric irritation.

Selected product options

Anadin paracetamol capsules

Aspro Tablets (aspirin 320 mg)

Calpol Suspensions (paracetamol-based)

Cuprofen Tablets (ibuprofen-based)

Disprin Direct Tablets (aspirin) 300 mg

Disprol Suspension (paracetamol-based)

Hedex Ibuprofen Tabelts

Hedex Paracetamol Tablets

Inoven Capsules (ibuprofen-based)

Junior Suspension (ibuprofen-based)

Medinol Suspension (paracetamol-based)

Nurofen Tablets (ibuprofen-based)

Pacifene Tablets (ibuprofen-based)

Panadol Suspension (paracetamol-based)

Panadol Capsules and Tablets

Paracets Tablets (paracetamol-based)

Phor Pain Tablets ibuprofen-based)

Proflex Tablets (ibuprofen-based)

Reclofen Tablets (ibuprofen-based)

Tramil Capsules (paracetamol-based)

 Sometimes patients may enquire about 'stronger' analgesic formulations

In such cases, a combination product or a soluble formulation may enhance the placebo effects. Examples of products which may be justifiable under such circumstances are

Nurofen Plus Tablets (ibuprofen + codeine)

Nurofen Soluble Tablets (ibuprofen)

Panadeine Tablets (paracetamol + codeine)

Paracodol Capsules or Tablets (paracetamol + codeine)

While aspirin and ibuprofen are not contra-indicated in asthmatic patients who are not sensitive to aspirin, caution is still required. Such patients may tolerate topical ibuprofen.

Analgesics (topical)

What is the difference between analgesics and anaesthetics?

Both types of agents provide pain relief and can arguably be called analgesics. Anaesthetic agents have a well-defined mode of action (see section on anaesthetics) and will interfere with all touch sensations. Smaller nerve fibres are, however, more sensitive to anaesthetic agents than to analgesic substances, with pain and autonomic impulses being preferentially blocked relative to coarse touch and movement.

Which compounds are available for topical analgesia?

A very wide variety of compounds are available for topical analgesia. However, these compounds can be conveniently grouped under salicylates, a series of NSAIDs or non-steroidal anti-inflammatory drugs (ibuprofen, diclofenac, felbinac, benzydamine, ketoprofen and piroxicam) nicotinates, capsaicin, and a miscellaneous group of agents of relatively little proven value.

How do topical analgesics work?

Salicylates, when administered orally, exert their analgesic activity by inhibiting the enzyme cyclo-oxygenase (see under analgesics (oral). Prostaglandin formation is thereby inhibited and pain relief follows. The extent to which this mode of action contributes to the overall activity of topical salicylates is unknown. However, it is known that salicylate esters are absorbed percutaneously and are hydrolysed by cutaneous esterases. Therefore, inhibition of prostaglandin synthetase is most likely a contributory factor to the perceived analgesia. This argument will clearly apply to the mode of action of ibuprofen and all other NSAIDs too.

The salicylate esters cause hyperaemia when applied to skin and it is claimed that they exert an analgesic effect by a counter-irritant effect, preferentially stimulating thick myelinated fibres during massaging and competing with pain signals for access to the pain integrating centre in the central nervous system. This competition for access to the pain evaluation centre is also postulated as a mechanism of action for the analgesia produced by warm or cold compresses and by cooling sprays. Topical analgesics are applied with massaging or rubbing and this is thought to ensure more rapid clearance of locally-produced pain-inducing substances (algogens).

Nicotinate esters cause vasodilation and increased clearance of algogens is therefore a possible mode of action for those compounds. Traditionally nicotinate esters are described as counter-irritants.

Capsaicin or its derivatives and capsicum extracts have come under much recent research interest due to the recognition that capsaicin is one of the most potent agents known for depleting nerve endings of substance P. Substance P, an undecapeptide exerts a wide spectrum of activity but in the present context, its pain-inducing activity when applied to peripheral sensory nerve endings is of most interest. Recent work indicates that capsaicin is effective in relieving pain associated with herpes zoster (shingles). Benzydamine has some anaesthetic and anti-inflammatory activities. It is also reported to exert an analgesic effect by stabilizing cellular membranes and inhibiting prostaglandins. Until data are available on a comparison of benzydamine against the more traditional salicylate esters, benzy-damine-containing products should be regarded as second-line topical analgesics.

Heparinoid-containing formulations, menthol, camphor, thymol, histamine, turpentine and adrenaline are among a wide miscellaneous group of agents promoted for topical pain relief. Little data is available to support their effectiveness. Camphorated oil, once widely recommended as a topical analgesic is now obsolete because of its high toxicity which has led to a number of paediatric deaths from accidental ingestion.

Are topical analgesics safer than oral products?

Topical therapy localizes most of the drug to the affected areas whereas systemic therapy leads to distribution throughout the body. Therefore topical therapy should theoretically be safer, although occasionally systemic adverse side-effects have been reported to follow topical application of NSAIDs. While systemic adverse effects become less likely, local side-effects and in particular hypersensitivity reactions may be enhanced. Nonetheless, on balance for conditions in which topical analgesics are effective, this mode of administration should be the first choice if patient acceptance is obtained.

Are analgesic plasters worthwhile?

Two types of analgesic plasters are available. One type is formulated with salicylate esters and well-established topical analgesics while the other is formulated with belladonna extract. Products in the latter type probably work by a placebo effect. Whether the salicylate plasters are any more effective is unknown but there is at least some theoretical justification.

Is there any rationale in combining nicotinate esters with salicylate esters in topical analgesic formulations?

Combining nicotinate and salicylate esters is certainly common practice. Whether such combinations are rational is uncertain. One study showed that benzyl nicotinate enhanced the absorption of salicylate, an effect which should be beneficial. However, a more recent study indicates that aspirin interferes with the vascular effects of the nicotinate esters and may therefore exert effects antagonistic to those of the salicylate esters. The difficulty in assessing pain relief means that it is unlikely that data will be forthcoming in the near future to provide an answer to whether combining nicotinic acid and salicylic acid esters is rational or irrational.

Precautions and when to refer

 Avoid eyes and mucous membranes.

 Avoid extensive use in children.

 General recommendations when recommending analgesics for muscular pain:

Rubefacients relieve muscular pain. The massage action during application no doubt contributes to this effect, as does a placebo effect.

Topical NSAIDS are effective too, but no more so than nicotinate or salicylate-ester-based products.

Topical NSAIDS are preferable to rubefacients in the presence of tissue inflammation.

Topical NSAIDS are unlikely to cause systemic problems unless the patient is hypersensitive or excessively high doses are applied.

Selected product options

Excessive exposure to sunlight should be avoided after application of NSAIDS.

Algipan Cream	Radian B Spray	Fenbid Gel (ibuprofen)
Balmosa Cream	Radian B Rub	Ibuleve Gel (ibuprofen)
Cremalgin Balm	Ralgex Cream	Ibuleve Spray (ibuprofen)
Deep Heat Creams	Ralgex Sprays	Oruvail Gel (ketoprofen)
Deep Heat Spray	Samaritan Cream	Proflex Cream (ibuprofen)
Lloyds Cream	Transvasin Rub	Traxam Pain Relief
PR Spray	Transvasin Spray	(felbinac)

Anthelmintics

How common are intestinal helminth infections?

Intestinal helminth infections are often considered only as third world diseases. In medical and pharmaceutical syllabuses, such infections are relegated to minor coverage under tropical medicines. Yet every general practice doctor or pharmacist knows that helminth infections are by no means rare even in the UK. It has been estimated that about 40% of all children under 10 suffer from threadworm infestations. Nematodes are the commonest infective helminths seen in practice. Cestodes, of which the tapeworm is the best known, are rarer causes of infection. Of the nematodes, the roundworm (*Ascaris lumbricoides* – ascariasis) and the pinworm or threadworm (*Enterobius vermicularis*) are more commonly encountered than the hookworm (*Ancylostoma duodenale* and *Necator americanus*). In the United Kingdom threadwormss or pinworms are the only commonly seen helminths.

How are helminth infections acquired?

Pinworms or threadworms are acquired by ingestion of the ova which subsequently hatch in the small intestine. Gravid female worms move to the colon and rectum to lay their eggs. The eggs, reaching the anal area, are then available to restart the cycle by hand to mouth transmission or by hand to hand to mouth transmission. Contaminated food, drink, bed clothes, fomites and house dust may also act as a reservoir for the parasitic eggs. Roundworms are acquired in a similar manner. The eggs may be viable for up to 1 year after excretion by the human host. Transmission rates are particularly high in dense populations living under poor sanitation in agricultural areas. School children are particularly commonly affected, probably because of frequent hand to mouth contact.

Tapeworms are acquired by ingesting contaminated beef (*Taenia saginata*), pork (*Taenia solium*) or fish (*Diphyllobothrium latum*). Improved animal husbandry has meant that tapeworm infestation is now rare in Europe. Many of the cases which are seen are acquired by consumption of contaminated and undercooked meats in countries where the animals are commonly infected.

How dangerous are helminthic infections?

Roundworm and pinworm infections cause much alarm when identified by the young patient or parent. However, such infections are generally not serious since treatment is usually effective and complications of the disease are rare. The most serious complications are due (1) to migration of the worms to cause obstruction of the hepatic duct, appendicitis and pancreatic duct obstruction or (2) intestinal obstruction by a bolus of worms, leading to intestinal perforation. Failure to thrive may be observed in heavily infested children on poor diets.

Hookworm and tapeworm infestations are generally more serious than those due to roundworms or threadworms because treatment is less satisfactory and the diseases themselves may lead to potentially more serious complications. Megaloblastic anaemia is an important complication since the worm appears to have great avidity for vitamin B_{12} and folic acid. Cysticerci of the worm may settle in body tissues including the muscles causing fever, muscle pain and high eosinophilia. Cysts of the worm may cause bronchial blockage and intracranial and hepatic cysts may be lethal.

In the United Kingdom, only piperazine salts and bephenium hydroxynaphthoate have for a long time been available for non-prescription use for the treatment of pinworms and roundworms. More recently, mebendazole has been down-regulated for the two-dose non-prescription treatment of enterobiasis (threadworms) while pyrantel pamoate has been down-regulated for the single dose treatment of threadworms and roundworms.

Are there any precautions to be observed with the anthelmintic agents?

Piperazine has a long history of use in the United Kingdom and a number of adverse reactions have been reported to follow its use. The drug has been reported to precipitate *grand mal* attacks in patients with a history of epilepsy. For this reason, piperazine is not recommended in patients with a history of central nervous system pathology. The drug also exerts neurotoxic side-effects, including visual disturbance, vertigo and impaired consciousness, at high doses. At the normal recommended doses, in patients without a previous history of neurological abnormalities or renal disease, these complications are rare.

Piperazine may potentiate the extrapyramidal effects of the phenothiazines and concurrent use of piperazine and the phenothiazines should therefore be avoided. Piperazine has been associated with isolated cases of teratogenicity and the drug should therefore not be used in the first trimester of pregnancy. The excretion pattern of piperazine in breast milk is unclear and avoidance of the drug in the nursing mother is recommended until more information to show the drug's safety becomes available. The drug is largely excreted in the kidneys and therefore care is required in the presence of renal malfunction since cumulation in the blood may increase the likelihood of adverse effects.

Mebendazole is potentially embryotoxic and teratogenic and should therefore be avoided in pregnancy. The evidence is more reassuring with pyrantel pamoate but good practice nonetheless dictates caution. Little is known about the excretion of mebendazole and pyrantel in breast milk. Again medical supervision is recommended for such patients. Pyrantel pamoate is no longer marketed in the UK despite its recent down-regulation to P status.

How often should the anthelmintics be used for eradicating the worms?

For threadworms and roundworms, two single doses of piperazine, spaced 2 weeks apart, are usually recommended. Some manufacturers recommend further monthly single doses to prevent reinfection by the roundworm but this seems to be largely unnecessary. With threadworm infections, all members of a family with a known infected person should be simultaneously treated. For mebendazole, two single doses two weeks apart are the ideal regimen. Pyrantel is licensed only as a single dose treatment in the UK.

Should a laxative be recommended together with an anthelmintic?

In persons with normal bowel movements, a laxative is unnecessary during treatment with an anthelmintic. In the presence of constipation, a laxative may be helpful and one product (Pripsen) is in fact a combination of piperazine phosphate and sennosides.

Precautions and when to refer

(R) Hookworm and tapeworm infestations.

(R) Patients with a history of CNS pathology.

(!) Pregnant women.

(!) Nursing mothers. Leave at least 8 hours between dose and breast-feeding.

(!) Renal malfunction.

(!) Piperazine antagonizes pyrantel pamoate.

Antiperspirants

What causes perspiration?

Under resting conditions, the body loses about 600 ml of water per day, through the skin and the lungs. This imperceptible loss of water occurs irrespective of the body temperature. When the body temperature rises, a more efficient mechanism than diffusion through the skin comes into operation. This mechanism is sweating. Sweating provides a usually efficient and rapid method for body temperature control and it is sweat which is normally perceived as perspiration. However, under conditions of high ambient humidity, normally imperceptible transcutaneous diffusion of water may contribute to the perception of sweat. Sweating or perspiration originates from the eccrine sweat glands which are innervated by sympathetic cholinergic nerves although they are also responsive to circulating adrenaline and

Table 3 Drugs which may cause sweating.

Amiodarone	Lofepramine
Amitriptyline	Maprotiline
Bethanidine	Mazindol
Buprenorphine	Medroxyprogesterone
Clomipramine	Mianserin
Debrisoquine	Nalbuphine
Desipramine	Nefopam
Dexamethazone	Nortriptyline
Dextromoramide	Pentazocine
Diflunisal	Perhexiline
Disopyramide	Pericyazine
Dothiepin	Phenazocine
Doxapram	Phenelzine
Doxepin	Prazosin
Epoprostanol	Prednisolone
Etretinate	Ritodrine
Fenoprofen	Sodium nitroprusside
Fludrocortisone	Sulindac
Fluspirilene	Terfenadine
Hydrocortisone	Thyroxine
Imipramine	Timolol
Iproniazid	Tranylcypromine
Isocarboxazid	Trimipramine
Isotretinoin	Viloxazine
Levodopa	Vitamin K
Liothyronine	

non-adrenaline. Surprisingly, except for the sweat glands in the hands and feet which may have both adrenergic and cholinergic innervation, those in other parts of the body are free from adrenergic innervation.

When the body temperature rises through exercise or exposure to pyrogens, signals are conveyed to the temperature regulating centre in the hypothalamus and from thence to the sweat glands, although vasodilation and decrease in heat production are also important body temperature control mechanisms. With increased sweat gland activity, perspiration accumulates as output exceeds evaporative losses.

Can drugs cause excessive sweating?

Both cholinergic and adrenergic drugs may induce sweating. Surprisingly some drugs with anticholinergic activity may also produce the same effect, probably through a different mechanism. Table 3 lists drugs which have been claimed to be associated with perceptible sweating.

What is the composition of sweat?

Sweat usually refers to eccrine gland secretions. It is an essentially colourless liquid with a pH ranging from 4 to 6.8. Water makes up to 99% of the bulk. Potassium, magnesium, iron, copper, manganese and other metals are present in trace amounts. Sodium chloride is an important component and indeed chloride levels in sweat are used as a diagnostic aid for cystic fibrosis. Organic compounds found in trace amounts in sweat include ascorbic acid, citric acid, lactic acid and urea. Apocrine secretions, on the other hand, are more complex mixtures than eccrine secretions. Proteins, lipoproteins and lipids are major components.

How do antiperspirants work?

The only antiperspirants in common use are the aluminium compounds (aluminium chloride, aluminium chlorohydrates, aluminium zirconium chlorohydrates and buffered aluminium sulphate). Their mechanism of action is still unclear but obstruction of the sweat duct with feedback inhibition of sweat secretion is the most widely accepted theory. Aluminium chloride hexahydrate 10% in industrial methylated spirits was until recently available on a prescription-only basis. It reacts with sweat to produce a more acidic, and hence potentially more irritant, solution than the more widely used aluminium chlorohydrates.

What advice should one give to patients using Anhydrol Forte?

This product contains 20% aluminium chloride hexahydrate and is therefore potentially more irritant than the cosmetic brands of antiperspirants. It should not be used as an ordinary everyday antiperspirant. To minimise skin irritation, the product should only be applied to healthy, dry, unshaven and non-depilated skin. Only night-time use is recommended spaced at least one hour from bath-time. Concurrent use of other skin products should be avoided.

Do antiperspirants have deodorant properties?

The aluminium compounds have antibacterial, and hence deodorant properties. However, more commonly, conventional antimicrobial or antiseptic compounds are added to antiperspirant formulations to yield more effective deodorants.

Precautions and when to refer

 Excessive sweating with no obvious cause.

 Nocturnal sweating.

 Sweating in patients returning from malarious countries.

 Avoid contact with eyes and do not shave axilla or use hair removing products within 12 hours of use.

Branded products worth considering

(all based on aluminium compounds)

Anhydrol Forte	Fresh and Dry Spray	Soft and Gentle Spray
Arrid Cream and Roll-On	Mum Roll-On	Sure Roll-On
Body Mist Liquid and Spray	Norsca Roll-On	Sure Spray
	Norsca Spray	Three Wishes Spray
Body Mist Roll-On	Right Guard Spray/	Yardley Roll-On
Fresh and Dry Roll-On	Roll-On/ZR	

Antiseptics

How dangerous are common micro-organisms contaminating the home?

There is little doubt that bacterial contamination is common in both dry and wet areas of the home, although the wet areas (baths, basins, dish-cloths, toilets) are consistently more heavily contaminated. Potentially pathogenic organisms recovered in a recent study included enterobacteria, notably *Escherichia coli*, *Staphylococcus aureus*, *Pseudomonas aeruginosa* and presumptive salmonellae. Kitchen-sink waste traps and nappy soaking solutions were particularly heavily contaminated despite the use of disinfectants. It is surprising that the sink wastes were found to be more heavily contaminated than the toilet bowls.

Many of the micro-organisms recovered can potentially induce serious infections. To provide some perspective about relative risk, a recent study on a healthy volunteer showed that ingestion of 10^6 pseudomonas cells could be handled by the healthy human body without ill-effects. Despite the fact that household bacteria are unlikely to trouble the average householder, decontamination to low levels is still desirable to minimize the risk of infections in susceptible individuals.

Complete disinfection appears to be an impossible goal in practice. While disinfectants are useful they are largely inactivated in the presence of organic contaminants as are present in sink traps. Improved hygiene around the home appears to be the most positive approach. Nappy buckets should be emptied in the toilets rather than down the kitchen sinks. Dish cloths should be dried immediately after use. Cross-contamination between fresh and cooked foods should be avoided. After dish-washing a second clean flush may be helpful as is evidenced by the relatively low bacterial counts in the toilet bowls. When a disinfectant is used for surface decontamination, a hypochlorite-based product should be the first choice.

Which antiseptic proprietary product should one recommend?

The activity of medicinal compounds is highly sensitive to changes in formulation and this is particularly pronounced with topical antimicrobial substances. Inactivation of these substances by impurities is well known, as is their incompatibility with many excipients. It is therefore not possible just from an inspection of the antimicrobial agent present to assess whether any given product is superior in activity to another. Comparative data for the different products are necessary for making valid assessments but unfortunately such data are rarely available to the practitioner. Published studies have generally been limited in scope and generally do not provide a sufficient number of identified comparators for drawing practical conclusions. For example, in one study a 1% chlorhexidine solution in a detergent base was compared only with a 1% hexachlorophane soap. Such studies are more useful for brand managers promoting their products than for patients or their advisers. However, knowing which active agent is present in an antiseptic formulation is still useful since this will give some indication of any toxicological problems which may arise. Chlorhexidine, for example, is generally less toxic to tissues than are the phenolics.

Are alcohols useful as antiseptic or disinfectant compounds?

Ethanol, generally referred to as alcohol, and iso-propyl alcohol are commonly used as disinfectants. With ethanol, the denatured formulations, surgical spirits and methylated spirits are usually employed. For skin antisepsis, surgical spirit or colour-free industrial methylated spirits (IMS) is preferable to coloured mineralized methylated spirits in order to minimize the risk of contact hypersensitivity, although even with the neat alcohols the occasional contact allergy has been reported in the literature.

Ethyl alcohol has been shown to kill bacteria both *in-vitro* and *in-vivo*, probably by denaturing proteins. This activity also means that the alcohol is toxic to human cells and because of this the application of alcohol to open wounds is not recommended; 70% aqueous ethyl alcohol is better than pure alcohol in killing bacteria. The same also applies to isopropyl alcohol.

Alcohol is less effective against spores than against the vegetative forms of bacteria and because of this, both ethanol and isopropyl alcohol are no longer recommended for sterilizing surgical instruments.

Benzyl alcohol is used as a preservative in some pharmaceutical formulations but its activity is too slow for recommending its use as a surface antiseptic.

Is it true that some natural oils are antiseptic?

There is certainly some evidence to show that certain volatile oils are antiseptic. However, there is currently insufficient data to enable comparison of the natural antiseptic oils with more established antiseptic compounds such as chlorhexidine and cetrimide. There is therefore a need for manufacturers promoting antiseptic products based on the natural oils to substantiate their claims before their products can be recommended.

Do bacteria develop resistance to antiseptics?

Strains of a given micro-organism may show resistance to a concentration of an antiseptic that kills or inhibits the majority of other strains of that same organism. In that sense therefore resistance to antiseptics is well known. The mechanisms by which bacteria develop resistance to antiseptic agents, in contrast to antibiotics, is poorly understood. Except for resistance to mercuric ions, there is no strong evidence to suggest that resistance to any of the commonly used antiseptic agents is plasmid-mediated. Selection of specific strains appears to be the most likely route to development of resistance to antiseptics and organisms with an ability to prevent antiseptic penetration are often involved. In some cases, organisms selected out may be better able to metabolize the antiseptic agent than susceptible strains.

Should cutaneous abscesses be treated with topical antiseptics?

Topical antiseptics are unlikely to be useful in the management of abscesses because of poor delivery via the skin and because of the poor activity of most antiseptics against possible anaerobic micro-organisms present. In a recent study of specimens from over 200 cutaneous abscesses, about a quarter of the cases yielded pure cultures that were predominantly *staphylococcus aureus*. In the other cases, mixed infections with both aerobic and anaerobic organisms were involved. Among the aerobes were α and non-haemolytic as well as group A ß-haemolytic streptococci, *enterobacter* and E. coli. The predominant anaerobes were gram-positive cocci, *Bacteroides* species and *Fusobacterium* species.

How safe and effective are iodine antiseptic products?

Iodine is available in several formulations including Iodine Tincture BP, decolorized iodine tincture and povidone iodine solutions. All are safe provided adequate precautions are exercised in their use. Long-term use should be avoided as should application to extensive areas of the skin, particularly in the young, as iodine absorption has been reported to lead to levels sufficient to impair thyroid function. This is more likely if the skin barrier is damaged as in burns. Some authorities recommend that iodine products should be avoided in infants and pregnancy. Iodine products may lead to the occasional sensitivity reactions and some data suggest that concentrations of iodine above 0.1% may inhibit wound healing.

Iodine, when formulated either in the free state or as the polyvinyl pyrrolidone complex, is active against a variety of bacteria, fungi, protozoa and viruses. Spores may also be inactivated. Contamination of povidone-iodine solutions by *Pseudomonas cepacea* have been reported, thus showing that important limitations exist in the spectrum of activity of iodine formulations. In exerting its antimicrobial activity, iodine appears to have selectivity for the bacterial cytoplasm and the cytoplasmic membrane. As with most antibacterial substances with a high affinity for organic substances, the presence of such matter may lead to inactivation of iodine. Pus, fat, cornstarch, nonionic and ampholytic surfactants as well as blood constituents have all been shown to interfere with iodine's antimicrobial activity.

Precautions and when to refer

 Deep-seated or spreading skin infections.

 Persistent skin infections.

(!) Severe hypersensitivity reactions may occur to all antiseptic agents including chlorhexidine gluconate.

(!) Avoid iodine-containing antiseptics on broken skin.

(!) Avoid use of crystal violet particularly on mucous membranes.

(!) Avoid prolonged use in infants and pregnancy.

Selected product options

Acriflex Cream (chlorhexidine gluconate)
Aquasept (triclosan)
Brulidene Cream (dibromopropamidine)
Dettol Cream (tricolosan + chloroxylenol + edetic acid)
Dettol Fresh (benzalkonium chloride)
Drapolene Cream (benzalkonium chloride and cetrimide)

Hioxyl Cream (hydrogen peroxide) for leg ulcers and pressure sores
Savlon antiseptic cream (chlorhexidine gluconate)
Savlon wound wash (chlorhexidine gluconate)
Savlon Concentrated Antiseptic (chlorhexidine gluconate + cetrimide)

Asthma

What is asthma?

Asthma is a disease of the respiratory system characterized by bouts of breathing difficulties. Asthmatics suffer from increased responsiveness of the trachea and bronchi to a variety of stimuli. When challenged the patients react with narrowing of the airways, tightness of the chest and wheeziness. Characteristically, acute attacks are interspersed with often prolonged symptom-free periods.

The prevalence of asthma varies from country to country and in some countries close to 1 in 5 children are said to be affected. In the UK population as a whole a prevalence of 1 in 20 has been suggested. More worryingly the prevalence of the disease appears to be rising.

Are there any non-prescription remedies for asthma?

Theophylline-containing products, widely prescribed for asthmatics by British doctors, are available without a prescription. However, asthma should ideally be managed under medical supervision although pharmacists and other health-care workers can participate in monitoring asthmatic patients. Products containing *Datura stramonium* are still available as non-prescription asthma remedies. Since stramonium contains anticholinergic compounds there is some rationale in its use in asthma. Indeed the smoking of cigarettes containing *Datura stramonium* was first recommended to asthma patients over 100 years ago. However, much more effective and specific therapies including selective β_2 sympathomimetic agents, synthetic anticholinergics and steroids now make *Datura stramonium* obsolete.

Further references

See under coughs and colds.

Product options

None of the OTC products are worthwhile. Theophylline-based products are best taken with regular medical supervision.

Athlete's foot

What is athlete's foot?

Athlete's foot is a term commonly applied by patients to any rash occurring on the soles of the feet or between the toes. In the medical and pharmaceutical literature, the term is usually restricted to infections of the feet caused by fungi. The condition commonly affects sportsmen sharing communal wash places and hence the term athlete's foot. The technical term used for the condition is *tinea paedis* to distinguish it from *tinea capitis* (scalp infections by the same fungus), *tinea corporis* (ringworm affecting the body) and *tinea cruris* (fungal infections affecting the groin, perineum and anal region). Jock's itch is a term sometimes used for the latter as is Dhobie's itch. *Tinea unguim* is a fungal infection affecting the nails.

Which fungi cause athlete's foot?

Several taxonomically-related fungi, collectively referred to as dermatophytes, are known to be causes of athlete's foot. The most common are *Trichophyton rubrum*, *Trichophyton mentagrophytes* and *Epidermophyton floccosum*. Other micro-organisms such as *Candida albicans*, *Corynebacterium minutissimum* and pseudomonads may cause lesions similar to those seen in athlete's foot or may complicate dermatophytic infections.

What defence mechanisms are active against dermatophytic infections?

The skin itself provides an effective primary barrier against dermatophytic invasion. This barrier is however impaired by a high ambient humidity and by physical abrasion and cracks. Following a primary attack, an immune reaction is established and this provides additional protection against subsequent infections. This explains why individuals with athlete's foot eventually become completely immune to the infection although several reinfections may be observed before that stage is reached. Dermatophytic microorganisms do not normally invade deeper tissues and this is now thought to be largely due to unsaturated tranferrin which acts as a non-specific serum inhibitory factor. Specific immune responses involving the antibodies must also clearly contribute to the relative resistance of the body against systemic dermatophytic invasion.

What agents are available for the treatment of athlete's foot?

Several distinct types of active ingredients are used for the treatment of athlete's foot. Keratolytic agents, in particular salicylic acid, are still widely used for the relief of athlete's foot. The combination consisting of salicylic acid and benzoic acid (Whitfield's Ointment) has stood the test of time and is still widely prescribed although the antimycotic agents tolnaftate, chlorphenesin, undecylenic acid and its salts and the newer imidazole compounds (clotrimazole and miconazole) are now often preferred. Tannic acid, boric acid and their combinations are included in some formulations with the claim that tannic acid is a useful astringent for drying the lesions. Aluminium acetate lotion is also used for the same purpose and indication.

How do the antifungal agents work?

The acidic compounds (salicylic acid, benzoic acid and undecylenic acid) exert their antifungal activity by diffusing into the fungal cell in the non-ionic lipophilic form. Within the cell, the acids dissociate into the ionic form and shift the intracellular pH. The pH change if pronounced enough, inactivates the enzyme phosphofructokinase and leads to accumulation of fructose-6-phosphate. Adenosine triphosphate levels fall and fungal growth is inhibited. The acids will also stimulate keratolysis and hence more rapid shedding of infected stratum corneum. The imidazoles probably work by acting as toxic analogues of metabolites essential for fungal growth. Inhibition of uptake of purines, resulting from or leading to fungal cell membrane disruption has also been suggested. Alteration in the permeability of the microsomal membranes is also thought to be involved. Tolnaftate inhibits sterol biosynthesis and causes accumulation of squalene and inhibition of cell growth.

Which is the best product to recommend?

The imidazole antifungal agents are now widely regarded as being the better remedies for dermatophytic infections. Undecylenic acid, tolnaftate and Whitfield's Ointment are also effective. There is surprisingly little evidence for the effectiveness of chlorphenesin, iodine and boro-tannic acid complex which are in some of the most widely used non-prescription products for the treatment of athlete's foot. Semi-solid formulations are probably preferable to lotions and powders although there is little experimental support for this.

How should the topical antifungal agents be applied?

Washing of the affected feet in warm water will help shedding of the infected stratum corneum. The feet should then be dried and the medication applied to the affected lesions. Coverage of areas adjacent to the lesions is recommended since apparently healthy skin is often infected. Application of a spray or a powder to the whole foot may also provide additional prophylaxis against spread of the infection to the healthy skin. Treatment should be continued for at least 2 weeks after the lesions have cleared.

What advice should diabetics be given about foot-care when on holiday?

Stasis is one of the main problems leading to ulcer formation. Therefore during long journeys diabetics should be advised to walk around at regular intervals. To avoid injury, shoes should be worn whenever possible but new shoes should be avoided. Airing of the feet at intervals will avoid maceration. Emollients applied to the feet will ensure that they remain supple and less liable to cracks. Swellings, sores or signs of ischaemia should be attended to immediately and professional help sought when necessary.

Precautions and when to refer

(R) Diabetic patients (slow healing of lesions).

(R) Lesions affecting the nails (do not respond well to topical agents).

(R) Lesions which do not improve after regular treatment for 2 weeks.

(R) Cases presenting with marked weeping and/or pus (bacterial superinfection).

Product options

Canesten Cream	Daktarin Cream	Mycil Gold Clotrimazole
(clotrimazole)	(miconazole)	Cream
Canesten Spray	Daktarin Powder	
(clotrimazole)	(miconazole)	

Second-line products (Tolnaftate-based)

Mycil Athlete's Foot Spray   Scholl Athlete's Foot   Scholl Athlete's Foot Spray
Mycil Athlete's Foot Cream   Cream   Tinaderm Cream
Mycil Powder   Scholl Athlete's Foot
     Powder

Third choice products

Germolene Footspray (tricolosan + dichlorophen)
Monphytol Paint (alkyl esters of undecenoic acid + salicylate esters + chlorbutol)
Quinoped Cream (benzoyl peroxide + potassium hydroxyquinoline)
Valpeda Cream (halquinol)

Bunions

What is a a bunion?

A bunion or hallux valgus is a deformity of the foot characterized by lateral deviation from the midline of the great toe. The medial side of the head of the metatarsal is enlarged while the metatarsal heads are depressed. There is also loss of the longitudinal arch and deformity of the heel.

What causes bunion formation?

The precise causes of bunions are unknown. Ill-fitting shoes, heredity and joint pathology (rheumatoid arthritis and gout) are generally thought to be, at least, contributing factors.

What are the symptoms associated with bunions?

Pain over the medial aspect of the metatarsal head is common and the bursa overlying the metatarsal head is often inflamed. The displacement of the bones causes localized pressure and the formation of corns and calluses. When the inflammation is severe, hospitalization may be necessary.

How should bunions be managed?

The presence of deformities means that corrective measures, usually surgical interventions, are needed. However, in the absence of severe associated problems, surgery is not indicated. Instead, supportive insoles and surgical shoes may be advised. Ill-designed shoes should clearly be avoided and callosities attended to. All cases of bunions should ideally be referred.

Burns

Should antiseptic products be used for treating burns?

Except for the most superficial burns, restricted to small areas of the body, the management of burns involves extensive wound dressing and specialist handling. Therefore if there is any suspicion of damage to the deeper skin layers, then no cream or ointment should be applied until definitive treatment has been decided upon. For the minor superficial burn, by the time the patient seeks advice the burnt area is usually covered with blister fluid and indeed in a number of cases the blister would already have burst and crust formation would be evident. When the affected area is contaminated, removing contaminated tissues with plain water should be the initial step to be followed by application of an antiseptic product. Running water is preferable to ensure that friction does not compound the problem. Cetrimide, chlorhexidine and povidone-iodine are all widely used and are all acceptable although their comparative effectiveness has not been fully assessed.

Solution and cream formulations are easier to apply and may therefore be preferable to ointments which may also interfere with wound healing.

Precautions and when to refer

(R) All but the most superficial scalds.

(R) When secondary infection is apparent.

(R) When the face or palms are affected.

Product options

Acriflex Cream (chlorhexidine gluconate)
Brulidine Cream (dibromopropamidine isethionate)
Drapolene Cream (benzalkonium chloride + cetrimide)

Savlon Antiseptic Cream (chlorhexidine gluconate + cetrimide)
Savlon Antiseptic Wound Wash (chlorhexidine gluconate)
Savlon Dry (povidone-iodine)

Chilblains

What are chilblains?

Chilblains are itchy erythematous or purple swellings which result from excessive exposure of the skin to low temperatures. Fingers, toes, noses and ears are commonly affected sites. More recently, the thighs have been identified as common areas for chilblains in horse-riders in the early frosty mornings.

How should chilblains be managed?

Prophylaxis of subsequent attacks is the most beneficial measure. Loose warm clothing will prevent chilblains affecting the thighs. Both tight-fitting shoes and open-ended sandals should be avoided during cold weather. Immigrants from warm climates to the Northern European winters are apparently common chilblain sufferers. Peripheral vascular diseases should be excluded in patients prone to repeated attacks of chilblains. Vasodilators are used both orally (inositol nicotinate and nicotinic acid) and topically (nicotinic acid esters) and may give symptomatic relief to some patients. Unsupervised use of oral nicotinic acid is not advised because of potential hepatotoxicity.

The value of acetamenaphthone, a vitamin K analogue, is even less clear. Its use in patients undergoing anticoagulant therapy is contraindicated. The drug is not advised in patients suffering from peptic ulceration or receiving anti-hypertensive therapy. Allergic reactions to acetamenaphthone are also possible. A number of other drugs including histamine, acetylcholine and soap spirit are used in chilblain remedies with little proof of efficacy. These should no longer be recommended.

Precautions and when to refer

(R) Patients with lesions not associated with exposure to cold.

(R) Lesions which do not heal within a week.

(R) Diabetic patients.

(!) Avoid use of acetamenaphthone.

Product options

Unbroken chilblains
Balmosa Cream (methylsalicylate/capsicum oleoresin)

Blistered chilblains (antiseptic creams)
Acriflex Cream (chlorhexidine gluconate)
Brulidine Cream (dibromopropamidine isethionate)
Drapolene Cream (benzalkonium chloride + cetrimide)
Savlon Antiseptic Cream (chlorhexidine gluconate + cetrimide)
Savlon Antiseptic Wound Wash (chlorhexidine gluconate)
Savlon Dry (povidone-iodine)

Cholesterol

There seems to be much current interest in blood cholesterol control. Is this justified?

The evidence associating a high blood cholesterol concentration and major ischaemic heart disease is now quite strong. The supporting evidence includes both retrospective and prospective epidemiological data. For example, in a recent study of close to 8000 men, the group with a total blood cholesterol level of more than 7.2 mmol/L had three times the risk of men with less than 5.5 mmol/L, of developing ischaemic heart disease. Controlling blood cholesterol therefore appears worthwhile.

However, a number of confounding variables suggest that caution is required in the interpretation of the data. For example, it is known that there is an increase in blood cholesterol level with age. Therefore, this should be taken into account when deciding on whether a given blood concentration is abnormally high. Gender is also a confounding variable to be considered. A recent study also suggests that a low cholesterol level may be associated with an increased cancer risk but the significance of this finding has yet to be defined. Irrespective of those concerns, dietary management of hypercholesterolaemia is good advice although the reduction in cholesterol levels achievable by this means is only modest.

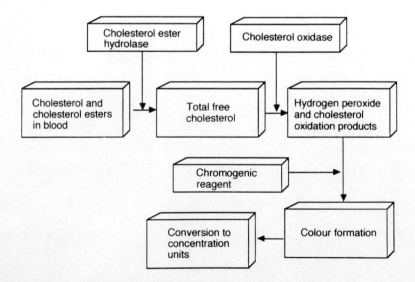

Fig. 2   Principles underlying current colorimetric assays for cholesterol.

How can cholesterol levels be measured?

A number of simple colorimetric tests are now available for measurement of blood cholesterol. Indeed a number of pharmacists and general practitioners now offer a cholesterol monitoring service. Campaigns by a number of associations interested in reducing cardiovascular disease are now carried out at regular intervals and blood cholesterol monitoring is often a feature of them. The biochemical basis for the tests is illustrated in Figure 2.

Is there any justification in having more extensive lipid profiles?

High density lipoprotein (HDL) levels are negatively associated with cardiovascular disease but how HDL protects against the disease is poorly understood. Despite this, it seems worthwhile to measure HDL cholesterol levels to obtain a more comprehensive assessment of the risk of cardiovascular disease and treatment options. However, measurement of total cholesterol should be sufficient in most cases. Serum triglyceride concentrations are not relevant to the prediction of ischaemic heart diseases.

Cold sores

What are cold sores?

Cold sores are lesions produced by the herpes simplex virus. For this reason, cold sores are commonly referred to as herpes simplex labialis. Cold sores are also called fever blisters.

What is the relationship between cold sores and genital herpes?

Both conditions are caused by the herpes simplex virus but different types are involved. With cold sores the type 1 virus, commonly referred to as HSV_1, is almost always the virus causing the lesion. At one time it was thought that genital herpes was only caused by the type 2 (HSV_2) virus but it is now known that HSV_1 is a common isolate from genital lesions particularly in individuals practising orogenital sex with partners infected by HSV_1. Surprisingly the buccal cavity and orolabial mucosa seem very resistant to infection by HSV_2. The reason for this difference is not known.

Are sites other than the lips and genitals affected?

Yes, the nose, the buccal cavity, the pharynx, the cervix, the intestines and the cornea are all potential sites of infection by the herpes simplex virus. Central nervous system infection is particularly dangerous while herpetic corneal infection is one of the commonest causes of blindness in the western world. Herpetic infection of the nail bed is known as herpetic whitlow and is a condition more commonly associated with nursing and medical staff than with the general population.

Is it true that the labial lesions are secondary sites of infection?

This is indeed a widely held theory. The initial infection is thought to occur primarily in the oropharyngeal cavity. However, primary lesions also occur on the lips.

Why do some individuals suffer from recurrent cold sores?

Recurrence is a feature of cold sores. The reason for this is that following the primary attack the virus is not usually eradicated. Instead some virus particles retreat into the nerve roots and lie dormant until reactivated by trigger factors. Why recurrence of lesions is seen in some individuals but not in others is not fully understood and currently the best explanation is normal variability of the efficiency of the immune system in different individuals. Specific immunoglobulins against the HSV_1 can be detected in the saliva of infected individuals but this seems to be inadequate to prevent reinfection in many individuals.

What are the most common trigger factors?

Sunlight or ultraviolet light, other infections, general ill health, inclement weather, some topically applied drugs such as 5-fluorouracil and physical abrasions are commonly identified trigger factors. Table 4 lists drugs which may reactivate herpes simplex or induce herpes simplex-like lesions.

Table 4   Drugs which may reactivate herpes simplex or induce herpes simplex-like lesions.

Drug		Cause
Cytotoxics most notably 5–fluorouracil		Reactivation of herpes simplex
Isoniazid		Vitamin deficiency and resultant labial or perilabial lesions
Acetarsol	Griseofulvin	Fixed drug eruptions
Acriflavine	Hydroxyurea	
Amidopyrine	Isoaminile citrate	
Amoxycillin	Meprobamate	
Ampicillin	Methaqualone	
Amylobarbitone	Metronidazole	
Arsenicals	Minocycline	
Aspirin	Nystatin	
Atropine	Oxyphenbutazone	
Barbiturates	Paracetamol	
Bisacodyl	Penicillins	
Buthalitone	Phenacetin	
Butobarbitone	Phenazone	
Carbromal	Phenobarbitone	
Chloral hydrate	Phenolphthalein	
Chlordiazepoxide	Phthalylsulphathiazole	
Chlormezanone	Quinine	
Chlorphenesin carbamate	Salicylates	
Codeine	Succinylsulphathiazole	
Co-trimoxazole	Sulphadiazine	
Cyclizine	Sulphadimethoxine	
Dapsone	Sulphadimidine	
Dicyclonine	Sulphamerazine	
Dimethylchlortetracycline	Sulphamethoxazole	
Diphenhydramine	Sulphamethoxydiazine	
Dipyrone	Sulphamethoxypyridazine	
Disulfiram	Sulphaphenazole	
Emetine	Sulphathiazole	
Erythromycin	Sulphobromophthalein	
Glutethimide	Trimethoprim	

How long does the infection last?

A cold core episode in patients suffering from recurrent infections typically starts with a prodromal stage characterized by itching and pain. This stage, which lasts for about 2 days, then develops into an active period of about a further 2 days during which lesions develop and virus shedding is at its highest level. Pain is also most intense during this period. Thereafter the condition subsides rapidly, viral titre declines exponentially and within the next 7 days most lesions should have healed completely.

How infectious is herpes simplex?

There is little doubt that genital herpes (infection) is highly infectious and is readily transmissible during sexual contact. There is much less information on the infectivity of labial herpes but it is unlikely to be any less than genital herpes. However, close contact again appears necessary.

How serious are herpes simplex infections?

Both types of infections are usually not dangerous although the associated discomfort can be intense. In a few groups of individuals, notably the newborn and immuno-compromised (e.g. patients on cytotoxic therapy), complications can be severe and dissemination of the disease extensive and life-threatening. Attempts to minimize exposure of these patients to the virus must therefore be made. Eczematous patients should also minimize the risk of infection as the infection can be severe in such patients.

Is there any cure for herpes simplex?

On current evidence it would appear that all existing therapies are inadequate and not curative. This is not because the available agents are not virucidal but because they cannot effectively reach the viruses as these retreat into the nerve roots or ganglia. Acyclovir is perhaps the most effective antiherpetic (HSV) agent in regular clinical use. Parenteral therapy is consistenly more effective than topical therapy in herpes simplex infections; indeed the magnitude of effect of topical acyclovir in cold sores is marginal (see below). Idoxouridine seems to be ineffective for HSV but is useful for herpes zoster infections (see shingles).

Are any of the non-prescription products effective?

It is possible that some of the products currently available may help in aborting attacks of cold sores and some may shorten the duration of the condition. However, only topical acyclovir (aciclovir) has been thoroughly tested. Evaluation of the effect of anti-HSV medications is particularly difficult because by the time the patient complains to the doctor or pharmacist the lesions are normally well on their way to complete resolution. This partly explains the very high placebo response rates of up to 80% reported in the literature to various ineffective treatments. Despite lack of curative attributes, many non-prescription products are helpful in alleviating the discomfort associated with the condition. Table 5 lists some substances claimed to be effective for herpes simplex but for which little supporting data is available.

Table 5   Substances other than acyclovir claimed to be effective for herpes simplex type 1.

Adenine arabinoside (POM)	2-deoxy-D-glucose	Lysine
Alcohol	Ether	Povidone-iodine
Chloroform	Idoxuridine (POM)	Silver sulphadiazine (POM)
Dimethyl sulphoxide	Lactobacillus	Vitamins

What is the mechanism of acyclovir's anti-viral effects?

On entry into the virus-infected cells, the drug is converted to acyclovir triphosphate by the herpes-specific enzyme thymidine kinase and host cell enzymes. The triphosphate then competes with deoxyguanosine triphosphate for incorporation into viral DNA thereby interrrrupting viral replication.

Is acyclovir cream useful for aborting cold sore lesions?

There is some evidence to support the claim that acyclovir cream applied at the first onset of the prodromal symptoms is effective in aborting cold sore lesions. Total healing time may also be shortened by a day or so but not all studies have yielded consistent results. It is worthwhile to note that once lesions have formed, topical acyclovir is of little value. It produces no decrease in pain or itch and the infection is not shortened. Therefore while acyclovir is of undoubted value in a number of viral infections, its efficacy as a topical cold sore product is only marginal.

Should we be concerned that topical use of acyclovir may lead to viral resistance?

Resistance to acyclovir has been shown to develop in-vitro. Except in immuno-compromised patients, there is no evidence that use of topical acyclovir leads to drug resistance.

Given that acyclovir is no panacea in cold sores, what additional advice should one give to cold sore sufferers?

Avoidance of trigger factors is important. Since ultraviolet radiation is a well-known trigger, use of a sunscreen with total sun-block properties prior to sunbathing should be recommended to known recurrent sufferers.

Precautions and when to refer

(R)   Patients on cytotoxic agents.

(R)   Infants.

(R)   Lesions persisting for more than 2 weeks.

(!)   Painless lesions (cancerous lesions may be painless).

(!)   Recommend that patients avoid exposure to neonates.

(!)   Check whether lesion could be drug-induced (this may be likely if cold sore associated with rashes elsewhere).

Product options

Blisteze Cream (ammonia + phenol)
Brush Off Cold Sore Lotion (povidone-iodine 10%)
Lypsyl Cold Sore Gel (lignocaine hydrochloride + zinc sulphate + cetrimide)
Zovirax Cream (acyclovir)

Colic

What is colic?

Infant colic is characterized by frequent episodes of irritability, forceful crying and fussing in an otherwise healthy and well-fed infant. The cause of infant colic is poorly understood but gaseous distension is often put forward as a cause of the cramps and spasms which the baby apparently suffers from. Stress appears to exacerbate infant colic and some authorities in fact believe it is causative. Hypersensitivity to certain foods ingested by the infant or the breast feeding mother has also been suggested as a possible cause of infant colic.

How should colic be managed?

The infant with colic often appears inconsolable and will only stop crying when totally exhausted. Such episodes are emotionally extremely demanding on the parents and they will need much patience at times of high stress. Deflatulent mixtures (simethicone) and carminatives may be useful placebos for the parents and may occasionally help the infant too. Sedatives (promethazine) should be avoided as should analgesics. The parents should be advised to give the baby frequent cuddles at times when colic is absent. This may help reduce stress and promote child–parent bonding.

Precautions and when to refer

- **(R)** Infant who fails to thrive.

- **(R)** Clearly exhausted parents.

- **(!)** Avoid alcohol-containing carminatives or gripe waters.

- **(!)** Avoid antihistamines and analgesics.

Products options

Dentinox colic drops (simethicone)
Infacol drops (simethicone)
Nurse Harvey's Mixture (sodium bicarbonate)

Woodward's Gripe Water (sodium bicarbonate; dill seed soil)

Common cold

What is the common cold?

The symptoms of the common cold familiar to all include rhinorrhoea, soreness of the throat, nasal congestion, hoarseness, cough and some degree of irritability. These symptoms are caused by infection of the upper respiratory tract by a variety of common cold viruses. Unlike influenzal attacks, with the common cold, fever and severe malaise are usually not accompanying symptoms.

Do children suffer from the common cold more often than adults?

Yes they do, except for a sharp drop in incidence during the first year of life. Pre-school children have the highest frequency. An incidence of five attacks each year is common. By the age of 10, the rate of common cold infections drops to about half that of pre-school children.

Do breast-fed babies have a lower incidence of common cold than bottle-fed babies?

Intuitively and based on the well-known protective effects of the immuno-protective components of breast milk, one would expect this to be the case but there has as yet not been any rigorous study to test whether this is indeed so. There is also no reason to contraindicate breast-feeding in the presence of the common cold in either mother or sibling.

What factors, other than exposure to the viruses, predispose to the common cold?

Stress and smoking appear to increase susceptibility to the common cold as does general ill-health. Exposure to a low temperature does not by itself lead to colds. Deficiency in vitamin C depresses the immune function as does malnutrition in general. However, despite claims to the contrary additional vitamin C or vitamins beyond daily requirements do not increase resistance to the common cold.

Can a person catch a cold several times in one season?

There is indeed no reason why a person cannot catch colds several times in succession. Immunity to one virus does not confer immunity to others. Therefore although a common cold episode is followed by at least transient immunity to the virus or viruses involved, other viruses can initiate fresh attacks. Relapses are of course also possibilities. The rhinoviruses alone exist in more than 100 serotypes.

How is the common cold transmitted?

Most cross-infections are probably the result of physical contact. Hand to hand transmission and hand to object transmission are perhaps the commonest routes. Airborne spread through droplets produced by sneezing and coughing is a further but less important mode of transmission of the common cold.

What is the natural course of a common cold?

Symptoms usually resolve within 1–2 weeks. In adults the 1-week long episodes are commoner while in the young attacks lasting 2 weeks are not uncommon. In some children the common cold is complicated by asthma-like wheeze. Resolution of symptoms may then be more prolonged. Exacerbations of symptoms of chronic bronchitis may be observed in adults.

How should common colds be managed?

Symptomatic relief is the most logical approach since effective antiviral compounds against the common cold viruses are not yet available. Interferons held much promise as effective non-specific antiviral compounds. However, despite much effort, the best method of delivering and using interferons has yet to be established. Reports of success for interferons in the management and prevention of common colds have so far been modest.

Symptomatic relief may be directed at (1) rhinorrhoea, (2) cough, (3) nasal congestion, (4) pain and (5) fever.

Rhinorrhoea or the runny nose may be helped by antihistamines which through their anticholinergic activity reduce nasal secretory activity. However it is arguable whether suppression of secretions is desirable since most patients find congestion more unbearable than rhinorrhoea.

More recently, the anticholinergic drug ipratropium bromide has been evaluated, in the form of a nasal spray, for the control of rhinorrhoea. Early results are promising but it is doubtful whether patients will actually prefer such a product to others currently available for the symptomatic relief of the common cold.

Nasal congestion follows rhinorrhoea in most common cold attacks. Sometimes it appears as the first symptom. Either way, nasal congestion is a symptom of local oedematous nasal tissues which interfere with free-flow of air and secretions. The oedema itself results from cellular damage and tissue hyper-permeability caused by viral attack and the release of mediators of inflammation and permeability. Decongestion may be achieved by topical or oral decongestants.

Pain and fever will be relieved by paracetamol. Aspirin is now no longer recommended for use in the paediatric population and indeed product licences for all paediatric aspirin-containing formulations have been withdrawn in the United

Kingdom because of the reported association between aspirin ingestion and Reye's syndrome. This is a rare but potentially life-threatening encephalopathy associated with fatty changes of the liver. Even in adults the case for aspirin for relieving pain, headache or fever associated with the common cold is now debatable since Reye's syndrome has also been described in adults and paracetamol is an adequate alternative. In the previous edition of this book, we indicated that there was little justification for the use of ibuprofen instead of paracetamol in the common cold. With the wide experience we now have of the safe use of ibuprofen on a non-prescription basis, we are now of the view that ibuprofen is a good alternative to paracetamol in the common cold, for otherwise healthy individuals. The usual precautions about hypersensitivity to ibuprofen apply.

How does nasal congestion develop?

The permeability of the capillary walls within the nasal cavity are normally such that a steady state exists between the luminal fluids and fluids in the surrounding tissues. In the presence of immunological challenge by allergens such as pollen grains or invasive agents such as common cold viruses, cellular damage follows with the release of vasodilator substances and of other tissue toxic components including 5-hydroxytryptamine and histamine. The resulting increased permeability of the vascular walls leads to a net movement of fluids and polymorphonuclear cells into the surrounding tissues. Oedema is the observable end point and is perceived by the patient as nasal congestion.

Are volatile oils and compounds such as menthol useful for the relief of the common cold?

Most users of volatile oil-containing rubs and inhalants know that such products provide effective decongestion of the blocked nose. The volatile oils also have antimicrobial activities. Whether these properties of the volatile oils and compounds such as menthol help to shorten the duration of the common cold is not known. Recent work suggests that many of the oils have much more complicated activities than previously thought. Menthol for example has been shown to be a calcium channel inhibitor.

Are combination products containing decongestant, paracetamol, antihistamine and cough suppressants justifiable for the common cold?

They are certainly convenient and economical for the patient suffering from all of the common cold symptoms. However, there is little justification for their use in patients who are only troubled by a single symptom and proper advice by the pharmacist or general practitioner is necessary.

How safe are the common cold remedies?

For most patients the common cold remedies present no hazard. However, in some patients great care is required before administering oral sympathomimetic decongestants. The hypertensive patient and those on monoamine oxidase inhibitors are at particular risk of developing hypertensive crises. Infants have been reported to show symptoms of central nervous system excitation including nightmares and sleeplessness after oral ingestion of common cold remedies containing sympathomimetic decongestants. The US Food and Drug Administration has recently proposed that an additional warning about the danger of exceeding the recommended dose be put on products containing phenylpropanolamine because of the increased risk of haemorrhagic stroke.

What are sympathomimetic agents?

Sympathomimetic agents are substances which produce effects similar to those of impulses conveyed by the adrenergic post-ganglionic nerve fibres of the sympathetic system. With decongestants, the effect mimicked is vasoconstriction. Currently used sympathomimetic decongestants include phenylpropanolamine, phenylephrine, ephedrine, pseudoephedrine, naphazoline, oxymetazoline and xylometazoline. Each has different selectivity for adrenergic receptors as shown in Figure 3.

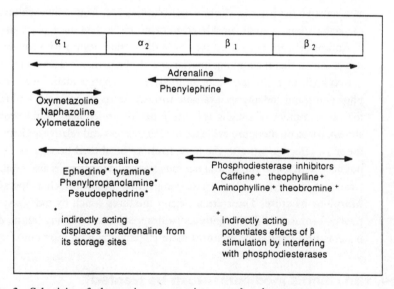

Fig. 3 Selectivity of adrenergic vasoconstrictors used as decongestants.

Are topical decongestants safer?

Topical decongestants are less likely to induce systemic adverse reactions and in this sense are therefore safer than orally administered sympathomimetic agents. Rebound congestion has however been reported following their use. Rebound congestion is commonly referred to as rhinitis medicamentosa. This is defined as the temporary increase in nasal congestion which is apparent as the vasoconstrictor effect of the nasal decongestants wears off. Secondary vasodilatation is thought to be the cause and on inspection a hyperaemic, oedematous nasal mucosa is observed.

Histopathological studies in animals suggest that rebound congestion is accompanied by an initial goblet cell (mucus secreting) hyperplasia, squamous metaplasia, local oedema, and destruction of cilia. Histochemical studies have confirmed the increased secretory activity and not surprisingly since this is associated with the mode of action, there is also evidence for a disturbed vasomotor response. The short-acting decongestants are particularly prone to inducing rebound congestion. Therefore, the longer-acting alternatives, xylometazoline and oxymetazoline should generally be preferred. Even then twice daily instillations for no longer than a week at a time are recommended.

The use of cough suppressants and expectorants for the common cold is the subject of many publications. In practice most practitioners succumb to the pleas of patients and recommend cough or expectorant mixtures. Some try even harder and recommend combination linctuses containing both expectorants and antitussives. This practice is often taken by cynics as evidence that neither antitussive nor expectorants are effective.

There is indeed little evidence to show that commonly used expectorants are active. Even with guaiphenesin, the most highly regarded expectorant, the evidence for effectiveness is equivocal. However, they no doubt make a useful contribution as a sedative for parents, doctors and pharmacists. Ammonium chloride and ipecacuanha are now often considered to be no more than mere placebos.

Antitussives are considered further in the section dealing with coughs. Generally it is accepted that if coughing interferes with the patient's sleep and if the cough is paroxysmal, then the use of an antitussive is recommended. Dextromethorphan, pholcodine and codeine are available without prescription in the United Kingdom for the treatment of coughs and the order of preference should probably be as shown, based on literature evidence of effectiveness and relative toxicity. Codeine is the most effective but also the most likely to be abused because of its more pronounced activity on the central nervous system. Morphine is also available for the treatment of coughs in the form of compendial products such as Ipecacuanha and Morphine Mixture. These are inelegant mixtures which by today's standards are poorly formulated. Their continued widespread use is baffling but no doubt some patients find unpleasant mixtures more effective than pleasant ones.

How can rhinitis medicamentosa be treated?

Simple abrupt or gradual discontinuation in the use of the offending vasoconstrictor is effective but not readily acceptable to the patient. Discontinuation of use, initially in one nostril, is more likely to be complied with. Oral decongestants are also an effective alternative if they are not otherwise contraindicated but they should not be used as an alternative to topical vasoconstrictors. Physicians have successfully used topical steroid sprays to wean patients off nasal vasoconstrictors. Explaining the nature of the problem to patients is generally regarded as helpful.

Is it true that nasal decongestants may cause hallucinations?

There is indeed some evidence that nasal decongestants and sympathomimetic agents in general, may cause hallucinations in a small proportion of children. In 1984, for example, the Committee on Safety of Medicines reported having received details of 16 cases of hallucinations in young children. While it is difficult to decide on whether the hallucinations were induced by fever or by the drugs ingested, current opinion is that in at least some patients the problem was probably iatrogenic. Although pseudoephedrine was claimed to be responsible for the hallucinations in the reports, literature evidence suggests that all sympathomimetic agents, both topical and oral, may exert the same effect.

What is the possible mechanism of action for this effect?

Hallucinations are in general poorly understood. However, as central nervous system manifestations, sympathomimetic agent-induced hallucinations are not difficult to rationalize. The sympathomimetic agents used as nasal decongestants possess structures very similar to the CNS active amphetamines (see Figure 4) and they would be expected to stimulate the same receptors once access to the brain has been gained.

Should bed-rest be recommended?

Influenzal attacks often debilitate patients sufficiently to require bed-rest. With the common cold patients are usually in good form otherwise and unless symptoms are severe there is little justification for keeping away from work or school. Although the common cold may remain infectious throughout its duration, opportunities for transmission early during the development of the cold would normally be sufficient to cross-infect any susceptible workmate or classmate. Excessive attempts to prevent cross-infection are not required since the disease is usually of no consequence except for inconvenience. There is no good evidence to show that common cold attacks are less common in groups showing high absenteeism. However, washing hands at regular intervals and after sneezing or nose-blowing should be recommended. With influenza and other viral infections, but not usually with the common cold, a post-viral fatigue syndrome may be observed after the acute stage (see later).

Is there any evidence that viral infections may also impair ciliary activity?

Recent work shows that infection by several of the common respiratory infections can lead to ciliary abnormalities in the nasal cavity. Therefore, in attributing ciliary damage to topically applied drugs, care must be taken to dissociate virus-induced from drug-induced damage.

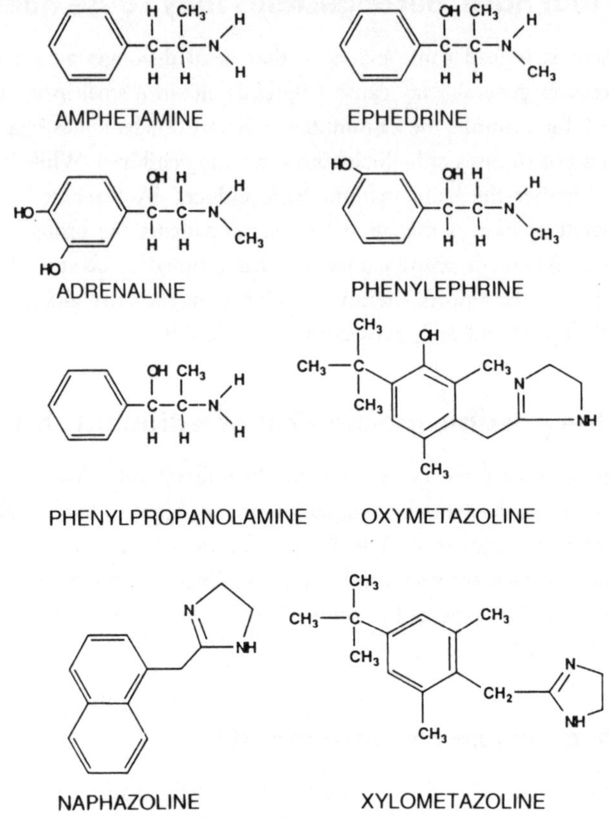

Fig. 4   Structure of sympathomimetic agents and amphetamine.

How can one distinguish influenza from the common cold?

Isolating and identifying the causative virus is obviously the most effective method. However, this is not as easy as it sounds and the approach is generally of little practical relevance. Influenza generally produces more serious symptoms than the common cold viruses and in practice the presence of a high temperature, marked lassitude and weakness are often used to indicate flu rather than the common cold.

Why are influenza vaccines commercially available while vaccines for the common cold are not?

Influenza is potentially a more serious infection than the common cold and the risk-benefit ratio therefore favours the influenza vaccines. In addition, fewer types of viruses are involved with influenza than with the common cold. The usefulness of vaccinating against influenza is therefore higher than vaccination against the common cold.

How many types of influenza are there?

Three antigenically distinct types – A, B and C – of viruses cause influenza. Influenza B is confined to man while influenzae A and C are also found in other animals. In man influenza A is the most important of the three viruses because its antigens change frequently and often abruptly and resistance to it is particularly transient.

How do influenza epidemics develop?

The viral antigens undergo constant change. Normally such changes occur slowly, a phenomenon referred to as *antigenic drift*, and most individuals are able to cope with such challenges. Occasionally, for unknown reasons, abrupt and large changes occur (*antigenic shift*); few individuals are able to withstand the new strain and an epidemic develops.

Who should be vaccinated against influenza?

Influenza vaccinations are recommended for individuals who are likely to develop serious complications of infection. Government health agencies therefore often recommend vaccinations against influenza for those with chronic lung disease, heart disease, renal disease and diabetes and for those being considered for immuno-suppressive therapy.

Some tissues are claimed to be virucidal. Are they effective?

The 'claimed' virucidal tissues are being promoted for reducing the spread of the common cold. Since transmission of the common cold commonly occurs by hand to hand to mouth or nose contact, the use of any disposable tissue would help reduce transmission of the viruses involved. The claim that addition of malic acid, citric acid and sodium lauryl sulphate to the tissues reduces transmission of the viruses more effectively than ordinary tissues has yet to be adequately supported.

What is lung-surfactant?

Lung surfactant is an alveolar lining layer with properties which permit surface tension control during breathing and hence normal lung function. The principal components of this so-called 'pulmonary surfactant' are phospholipids, notably dipalmitoyl phosphatidylcholine, phosphatidylinositol, lysolecithin, phosphatidyl ethanolamine and sphingomyelin. Lung surfactant has recently been the focus of attention in the management of respiratory distress syndrome, in the form of replacement therapy.

Why is persistent fatigue often a feature of convalescence from influenza?

No satisfactory explanation is currently available for explaining such post-influenzal fatigue. In fact such fatigue appears to be associated with many different types of acute viral infections and the term 'post-viral fatigue syndrome' is often used to describe the condition. Myalgic encephalomyelitis is also an alternative term, commonly used for describing the same type of condition. Many authors are of the opinion that although the symptoms typically follow a flu-like illness, the viruses involved are not the usual flu or common cold viruses. The Epstein-Barr virus, for example, is thought to be responsible for as many as 20% of cases. Histological examination of muscle biopsies reveals scattered necrotic fibres while nuclear magnetic resonance studies indicate disturbed glycolytic pathways leading to rapid intracellular acidosis during exercise.

Precautions and when to refer

(R) Patients with signs of severe systemic disturbance, e.g. very high temperature, severe malaise.

(R) Children and the elderly with severe colds.

(R) Patients with earache.

(R) Patients with brown or pus-loaded sputum.

(R) Worsening colds lasting for more than 2 weeks and with persistent fever.

(R) Patients with severe colds and with a history of chronic respiratory disease (bronchitics, asthmatics, etc.).

(R) Patients with severe chest pain on coughing or of sudden onset (pleurisy).

(R) Patients with severe facial pain (sinusitis).

(!) Do not give aspirin-containing products to children under 12 (Reye's syndrome).

(!) Do not give decongestants to patients with a history of stroke.

(!) Avoid decongestants in hypertensive or heart-disease patients.

(!) Avoid use of decongestants in patients with thyroid disease or diabetes.

(!) Avoid decongestants in young children.

(!) Avoid initiating treatment with topical decongestants (decongestant habit very difficult to discard).

(!) Avoid decongestants in individuals with a history of CNS disturbance (CNS adverse reactions more likely).

(!) Patients presenting with cough only need to be interviewed to exclude drug, notably ACE inhibitor-induced, coughing.

(!) Avoid concomitant use of products with different decongestants.

(!) Avoid oxymetazoline in acute porphyria.

Products options

When fever or pain, nasal congestion and cough are present
Beechams All-in-One Syrup (guiaphenesin, paracetamol, phenylephrine)
Benylin 4 Flu Liquid (paracetamol, pseudoephedrine, diphenhydramine)
Benylin 4 Flu Tablets (paracetamol, pseudoephedrine, diphenhydramine)
Boots Day Cold Comfort Capsules (paracetamol, pseudoephedrine, pholcodine)
Boots Night Cold Comfort Capsules (paracetamol, pseudoephedrine, diphenhydramine)
Day Nurse Liquid (paracetamol, phenylpropanolamine, dextromethorphan)
Day Nurse Capsules (paracetamol, phenylpropanolamine, dextromethorphan)
Vicks Medinite Syrup (paracetamol, dextromethorphan, pseudoephedrine)

When nasal congestion is main complaint
Actifed Tablets (pseudoephedrine, triprolidine)
Afrazine Nasal Spray (oxymetazoline)
Bronalin Elixir (pseudoephedrine)
Contac 400 (chlorpheniramine, phenylpropanolamine)
Dimotapp Elixir (phenylephrine, phenylpropanolamine, brompheniramine)
Dristan Spray (oxymetazoline)
Olbas Pastilles (volatiile oils)
Otrivine Spray (xylometazoline)
Otrivine Menthol Spray (xylometazoline)
Penetrol Inhalant (menthol peppermint)
Sudafed Elixir (pseudoephedrine)
Sudafed Spray (oxymetazoline)
Sudafed Tablets (pseudoephedrine)
Tixylix Inhalant (volatile oils)
Triominic Capsules (phenylpropanolamine, pheniramine)
Vicks Inhaler (camphor, mentol)
Vicks Sinex Spray (oxymetazoline)

When nasal congestion and pain or fever present
Barum Cold Relief Capsules (caffeine, paracetamol, phenylephrine)
Beechams Flu-Plus Powders (Vitamin C, paracetamol, phenylephrine)
Beechams Hot Powders (Vitamin C, paracetamol, phenylephrine)
Beechams Powders Capsules (caffeine, paracetamol, phenylephrine)
Benylin Day and Night Tablets (paracetamol, phenylpropanolamine)
Catarrh-Ex Capsules (caffeine, paracetamol, phenylephrine)

Cold Relief Capsules (caffeine, paracetamol, phenylephrine)
Coldrex Tablets (caffeine, paracetamol, Vitamin C, phenylephrine)
Distran Tablets (aspirin, caffeine, chlorpheniramine, phenylephrine)
Hedex Powders (paracetamol, phenylephrine, Vitamin C)
Lem-Plus Powders (paracetamol, phenylephrine, caffeine)
Lemsip Powders (paracetamol, phenylephrine, caffeine)
Lemsip Capsules (paracetamol, phenylephrine, caffeine)
Lemsip Flu Strength Powders (paracetamol, pseudoephedrine, Vitamin C)
Lemsip Max Strength Powders (paracetamol, phenylephrine, Vitamin C)
Lemsip Menthol Extra Sachets (paracetamol, phenylephrine, Vitamin C)
Lemsip Original (paracetamol, phenylephrine, Vitamin C)
Lemsip Powder+ (ibuprofen, pseudoephedrine)
Mucron Tablets (paracetamol, phenylpropanolamine)
Nurofen Cold and Flu Tablets (ibuprofen, pseudoephedrine)
Sinutab Nightime (paracetamol, phenylpropanolamine, phenyltoloxamine)
Sinutab Tablets (paracetamol, phenylpropanolamine)
Sudafed Co Tablets (paracetamol, pseudoephedrine)
Tiogesic Tablets (paracetamol, phenylpropanolamine)
Vicks Action Tablets (ibuprofen, pseudoephedrine)

Conjunctivitis

What is conjunctivitis?

Conjunctivitis is inflammation of the conjunctival tissues caused by chemical irritation, allergies such as hay-fever, or infection. Effective management will therefore depend on the cause. Bacterial infections may benefit from the use of a suitable eye drop while hay-fever symptoms may be alleviated by systemic antihistamines.

What causes watering eyes?

Exposure to a smoky and irritant atmosphere often leads to watery eyes because of excessive production of tear fluid. Commonly, however, watering eyes are due to blockage of the nasolacrimal duct (Figure 5) by infection or nasal problems. In the elderly the ageing skin may well sag to such an extent that the nasolacrimal duct is no longer in alignment with tear flow (senile ectropion) and tear drainage is therefore impaired. Persistent watering of the eyes will need referral to exclude serious underlying pathology.

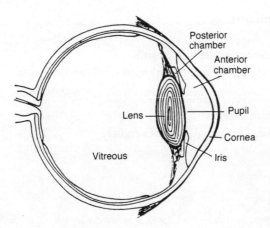

Fig. 5   Lachrymal apparatus of the eye.

What causes red eyes?

Excessive tearing is a well-known cause of a red eye. Another common cause is conjunctivitis, both of allergic and infective origin. Occasionally the red eye may be due to a subconjunctival haemorrhage. Discolouration is intense and although highly alarming to the patient, the condition usually resolves spontaneously within 2 weeks. More serious causes of the red eye include acute glaucoma, anterior uveitis and keratitis.

What is blepharitis?

Blepharitis is inflammation of the eyelids. The inflamed eyelids are red and scales are often seen sticking to the roots of the lashes. The condition is often chronic and is commonly associated with seborrhoeic dermatitis of the scalp. Treatment is often disappointing but management of the seborrhoea of the scalp often gives symptomatic relief in blepharitis.

Precautions and when to refer

(R) If vision is impaired.

(R) If infection does not clear within a week.

(!) Check for possibility of hay-fever.

(!) Avoid sympathomimetic eye drops containing phenylephrine or xylometazoline.

Product options

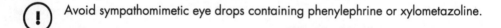

Allergic or seasonal conjunctivitis
Brol-eze Eye Drops (sodium cromoglycate)   Clearine Eye Drops (witch hazel, naphazoline)

Infective conjunctivitis
Brolene Eye Drops (propamidine isethionate)

Blepharitis
Brolene Eye Ointment

Eye Washes
Optrex Eye Drops (witch hazel)   Optrix Eye Lotion (witch hazel)   Refresh Eye Solution (polyvinyl alcohol)

Constipation

What is constipation and what causes it?

Constipation is defined as infrequent and painful evacuation of faeces. Normally it is the painful aspect of constipation which drives the patient to seek symptomatic relief, although in a number of patients a low frequency of stools is the more worrisome feature. A further subset of patients ascribe a variety of their ills to infrequent defaecation and therefore seek relief through laxatives. Constipation may be caused by a number of factors including poor dietary habits, loss of rhythm such as during travel, neglect of the urge to defaecate, impaired colonic motility often associated with the ageing process, constipating drugs and a variety of endocrinal conditions including hypothyroidism, pregnancy and diabetes mellitus.

Which are the constipating drugs?

A wide variety of drugs are potentially constipating. Examples include drugs with anticholinergic activity including the classical anticholinergics such as hyoscine and propantheline, the centrally-active antihistamines and the tricyclic antidepressants. Aluminium hydroxide, iron salts and opiates are other well-known examples. A more extensive but not exhaustive list is given in Table 6.

How should constipation be managed?

Constipation of sudden onset and/or alternating with episodes of diarrhoea needs referral. Chronic constipation not previously investigated to exclude underlying disease also needs referral, particularly if a change in severity is perceived. Initial therapy should involve a change in dietary habits to increase fibre intake and attempts should be made to persuade the patient to reinitiate regular motions by answering the urge to defaecate as soon as possible after it is felt. Regular physical activity is also said to help.

A change in breakfast cereals consumed from one of low fibre to one of high fibre content is relatively easy to adopt but may not be adequate to correct constipation. More fundamental changes in dietary habits may be more difficult to achieve and for this reason pharmaceutical bulking agents are helpful. Only when these measures fail should traditional laxatives be resorted to.

Food composition tables give crude fibre values. Are these the same as dietary fibre values?

The dietary fibre of plants is made up of a complex mixture of substances including celluloses, pectin, gums, mucilages and lignin. Crude fibre as listed in food

Table 6 Drugs which may cause constipation.

Aluminium hydroxide	Fenoprofen	Phenazocine
Amiloride	Fluphenazine	Phenelzine
Amitriptyline	Glipizide	Prazosin
Benorylate	Hyoscine butylbromide	Procyclidine
Benztropine	Imipramine	Promazine
Bromocriptine	Indomethacin	Propantheline
Chlorothiazide	Iproniazid	Ranitidine
Cholestryramine	Iron	Reserpine
Clomipramine	Isocarboxazid	Sucralfate
Clonidine	Levodopa	Sulindac
Codeine	Levorphanol	Trazodone
Colestipol	Lofepramine	Trifluoperazine
Desipramine	Maprotiline	Trimipramine
Dextropropoxyphene	Mazindol	Verapamil
Dicyclomine	Methixene	Viloxazine
Diethylpropion	Methyldopa	Vinblastine
Diflunisal	Morphine	Vincristine
Dihydrocodeine	Nortriptyline	Vindesine
Dothiepin	Papaveretum	
Doxepin	Pargyline	

composition tables, refers to the residue left after strong acid and base hydrolysis of the plant material. Crude fibre and dietary fibre are therefore two distinct entities.

Which bulk-laxatives are commonly used?

Bran, a by-product of milled wheat, is known to most diet-conscious individuals. Bran has been shown to be useful in the treatment of constipation by producing softer, bulkier stools, normalising transit and relieving symptoms. Large particles of bran appear to be better than small particles and raw bran is better than cooked bran. *Psyllium* and *ispaghula* are both refined preparations derived from the epidermal layers of the ripe seeds of different species of the herb *Plantango*. Sterculia (Karaya) gum is an exudate from the tropical shrub *Sterculia*. Polycarbophil is a non-absorbable water-retaining polymer obtained by cross-linking polyacrylic acid with divinyl glycol. Methylcellulose and sodium carboxymethylcellulose are semi-synthetic products forming viscous solutions with water. Various viscosity grades are available. Table 7 lists the fibres present in the various laxative formulations on the UK market.

Which is the best fibre-based laxative agent available?

Dietary fibre is the non-absorbable portion of plant-derived foods. Being non-absorbable, it increases faecal mass and thereby stimulates reflex peristalsis. Therefore the bulkier the resulting faecal mass, for a given weight of fibre ingested, the better the results. Two characteristics of the fibre used determine the resulting faecal mass: its water-holding capacity and its usefulness as a substrate for colonic bacteria. Indeed recent data suggest that the latter may be the more important of the

Table 7   Quick guide to bulk laxatives.

Fibre	Product	Main polysaccharides	Note
Bran fibre	Natural Fybranta tablets Proctofibe tablets Lejfibre biscuits Trifyba powder	Arabinoxylans	Contain gluten and should be avoided in coeliac disease
Isphagula husk fibre	Fybogel granules Isogel granules Metamucil powder Regulan powder Vi-Siblin granules	Arabinoxylans	Contains sodium – Contains sucrose Contains sucrose –
Sterculia fibre	Normacol special granules	Galacturonhamnans	
Methylcellulose	Celevac tablets Celevac granules Cellucon tablets Cologel liquid		

two mechanisms. For example, pectin has a high water holding capacity (56.2 g/g) but is poor at increasing faecal bulk. Bran on the other hand holds little water (4.2 g/g) yet has a six-fold greater effect on faecal weight than pectin. Advertising material based on *in-vitro* water-holding capacities of bulking agents may therefore be misleading.

Unfortunately, comparative data on the commercially-available bulking agents do not appear to be available but data would suggest that natural fibres which can act as substrates for colonic bacteria are preferable to non-degradable synthetic polymers such as polycarbophil on a weight to weight basis. Gel-forming characteristics and viscosifying effects may impart other attributes to the products which are desirable in prevention of clinical problems such as blood sugar control, hypercholesterolaemia and even colonic cancer.

Why do fibre and laxatives sometimes fail?

In some severely constipated patients, fibre and laxatives sometimes fail to induce defaecation. Recent work suggests that such failures may be attributable to an inability of the patients to co-ordinate the pelvic floor muscles to achieve expulsion of rectal contents.

How safe are the bulk laxatives?

The commonly used bulk laxatives are generally quite safe. However, cases of allergy, with asthma-like symptoms, have been reported with psyllium. Intestinal obstruction has also been claimed to follow ingestion of unprocessed bran. Dried fruits, often recommended as a source of fibre in constipation, have also led to a number of intestinal obstructions, particularly if eaten unstewed. Elderly people with dentures are at particular risk. Zinc chelation by the phytate (inositol hexaphosphate) in bran is known to decrease the bioavailability of zinc and the faecal excretion of copper and magnesium increases with hemicellulose supplementation. Therefore, there is the possibility of a mineral deficiency state induced by a high-fibre diet, particularly among individuals relying on single sources of the essential minerals and among those who are verging on a deficiency state prior to fibre supplementation. Some elderly patients may well fall into this group.

Danthron (chryzazin)

Danthron is a synthetic chemical, structurally related to the sennosides, and has been one of the, commercially, most successful laxatives. The most widely used formulation in the UK was at one time a suspension containing danthron and poloxamer 188. Recent work has shown that danthron is carcinogenic in rodents and as a result danthron-containing products are now restricted to prescription use.

What precautions should be observed and what advice should be given when recommending bulk laxatives?

Bran-containing products should be avoided in patients suffering from gluten enteropathies and coeliac disease. Patients at risk of mineral deficiencies (e.g. the elderly) or on an already high phytate diet (e.g. immigrants from the Asian subcontinent) may require additional mineral supplementation if the fibre intake is increased. Patients susceptible to intestinal obstruction such as those with known oesophageal strictures and those suffering from dysphagia should ideally avoid an excessive high fibre intake. If fibre supplements are administered to those patients then formulations to be predispersed prior to ingestion should be recommended. Chewable tablets should also be avoided by these patients, particularly if edentulate. Flatulence may be a problem in the initial stages but patients can be reassured that this problem normally disappears with continuation of therapy. Bulk laxatives are slow-acting and up to several days may be required before benefits are perceived. Some rare patients may become allergic to the mucilages. All bulk laxatives should be taken with plenty of water and should not be taken immediately before going to bed.

How do non-bulk laxative agents work?

Traditionally, in addition to the bulk laxatives, laxative agents are classified as osmotic agents, irritant or contact laxatives, emollient laxatives and lubricant laxatives, as shown in Table 8, based on their presumed physico-chemical or gross pharmacological activities. With the availability of improved biochemical techniques to investigate their modes of action, a reclassification of laxatives has been suggested as shown in Table 9. However, because the biochemical investigations are still incomplete, the classification in Table 9 must be regarded as tentative. In

Table 8   Traditional classification of laxative agents other than bulk laxatives.

1. Contact or irritant laxatives	Anthraquinones
	Aloe
	Casanthranol
	Cascara
	Danthron
	Frangula
	Rhubarb
	Senna
	Bisacodyl
	Castor oil
	Phenolphthalein
	Sodium picosulphate
2. Osmotic laxatives	Epsom salts (magnesium sulphate)
	Glauber's salts (sodium sulphate)
	Glycerin
	Sorbitol
	Lactulose
3. Wetting agents	Dioctyl sodium sulphosuccinate
	Poloxalkol (poloxamer 188)
4. Lubricant	Liquid paraffin
5. Others	Glycerin suppositories

the following discussion chemically or physico-chemically similar laxatives will be considered together.

The anthraquinone laxatives

Anthraquinone laxatives are obtained from a variety of plant sources including *senna, aloe, cascara, rhubarb* and *frangula*. Danthron is a synthetic anthraquinone laxative which unlike the naturally-occurring anthraquinones, is a non-glycoside. Casanthranol is a purified extract of cascara sagrada with up to 10 times the potency of the standard extract.

The main active compounds of sennoside laxatives are the glycosidic stereo-isomers, sennosides A and B. They are prodrugs which are metabolized by colonic bacteria to produce the active compound rheinanthrone. Danthron is much less active than the sennosides, possibly due to metabolic breakdown to inactive compounds. Unlike the sennosides, systemic absorption takes place prior to colonic activity. As such, danthron is therefore a less attractive laxative than the sennosides. The anthraquinone laxatives depress fluid absorption in the colon (Table 8) and hence promote the formation of softer stools. In addition, the sennosides but not danthron, accelerate colonic transport, an effect which is partly inhibited by the prostaglandin synthetase inhibitor indomethacin.

Table 9 Biochemical modes of action of non-bulk laxatives.

	Inhibits Na$^+$/K$^+$ATPase	Stimulates adenylate cyclase

Anthraquinones
  Senna
  Cascara
  Danthron, etc.
	+	?

Bisacodyl	+	?
Castor oil	+	+
Dioctyl sodium sulphosuccinate	−	+
Phenolphthalein	+	−
Sodium picosulphate	+	−

Based on Ganginella P. & Bass P. (1978) *Life Sciences* **23**: 1001.

Diphenylmethane laxatives

Bisacodyl, sodium picosulphate and phenolphthalein are diphenylmethane derivatives. Bisacodyl exerts an effect, which can be inhibited by a local anaesthetic, on
the rectum and for this reason it is commonly referred to as a contact laxative.
Bisacodyl and sodium picosulphate are known to be prodrugs of the same entity,
bis-(p-hydroxy-phenyl) pyridyl-2-methane except that bisacodyl is activated by
endogenous esterases while in the case of sodium picosulphate, microbial esterases
are involved. Bisacodyl and phenolphthalein have been shown to inhibit Na$^+$/
K$^+$ATPase and can therefore be expected to produce a hydrophoric or water-
accumulating, effect in the colon. Sodium picosulphate no doubt shares this effect.
Castor oil is a prodrug of ricinoleic acid which exerts a laxative action by altering
fluid and electrolyte movement. Both inhibition of Na$^+$/K$^+$ATPase and stimulation of adenylate cyclase are involved. Ricinoleic acid also increases colonic activity
and mucosal permeability.

Surfactant compounds

Dioctyl sodium sulphosuccinate (docusate sodium) and poloxamer 188 are surface
active compounds which were initially thought to act physically by lubricating the
faeces and making the faecal mass more permeable to water. It is now known that
the mode of action of dioctyl sodium sulphosuccinate is much more complex and
cyclic-AMP-mediated anion and hence water transport may again be the main
mode of action.

Inorganic salts

Epsom (magnesium sulphate) and Glauber's (sodium sulphate) salts are generally thought to act by exerting a hyperosmolar effect, leading to water accumulation in the intestines. For this reason they are commonly referred to as osmotic laxatives. The fact that low doses of magnesium salts are effective suggests a more complex mode of action and the involvement of the intestinal hormone cholecystokinin has been suggested. Glycerin and sorbitol are also thought to act as osmotic laxatives.

Liquid paraffin

Liquid parafin is poorly absorbed and probably works by physically lubricating faecal material.

Lactulose

This is metabolized by bacteria to produce lactic acid and a combination of other poorly absorbed acids. These exert an osmotic effect and hence softening of stools. The lowering of pH produced by the acids may also cause contraction of the colonic muscle.

How should a non-bulk laxative agent be chosen?

The more drastic laxatives such as castor oil, bile salts and the unpalatable Epsom and Glauber's salts should probably no longer be used. Mineral oil may lead to faecal incontinence and should be avoided. There is also the risk that long-term use may lead to oil-soluble vitamin deficiency. Traces of polycyclic hydrocarbons also cause some concern because of their mutagenic potential. Recent work suggests that the paraffins are absorbed and accumulate in the lymph nodes, spleen, liver and adipose tissues of humans as well as of animals. Such accumulation is known to be toxic in animals and for this reason the Ministry of Agriculture, Fisheries and Foods has recently banned their use in foods. It seems prudent to avoid these oils in medicinal products too.

Danthron has been associated with carcinogenicity in rodents and should no longer be recommended, given the availability of better alternatives. Single-active products are to be preferred to multiple-component products. Phenolphthalein and anthraquinone laxatives are excreted into breast milk, although with the anthraquinones the levels are probably inadequate to cause distress in the infant. Phenolphthalein has been associated with a number of skin eruptions. The anthraquinones may cause discolouration of urine and of the colonic mucosa (melanosis coli) but these are of no clinical significance. Based on these observations, a sennoside laxative would appear to be the first choice non-bulk laxative. Lactulose, bisacodyl and sodium picosulphate are suitable second-line laxatives.

Is purging an effective method for weight control?

Many teenagers abuse laxatives and diuretics in the belief that purging will reduce calorie absorption and hence produce a weight loss. Recent work has shown that any calorie saving is negligible but there is a serious risk of inducing electrolyte imbalance by this practice.

What is the irritable bowel syndrome and are laxatives useful in treating it?

Irritable bowel syndrome (IBS) is diagnosed when no gastrointestinal disease can be identified to account for the typical symptoms of irregular bowel habit, abdominal pain and distension. The disease is generally ascribed to a disorder in gut motility but there is a significant psychological component. Constipation tends to alternate with loose stools. Therefore laxatives are not usually a sensible choice although most gastroenterologists consider a bulk laxative worth trying. Ispaghula appears to be more effective than bran. Antispasmodics such as alverine and in particular mebeverine (POM) may relieve pain. Enteric-coated peppermint oil capsules (Colpermin) appear to be more effective than placebo in relieving pain in the irritable bowel syndrome. Dicyclomine is effective but the incidence of anticholinergic adverse effects is high.

Is it true that constipation is worse at certain stages of the menstrual cycle?

Severe constipation is indeed often seen in young women and it has been reported that normal menstruating women show changes in upper gastrointestinal transit between the follicular and the luteal phases of the menstrual cycles. Since constipation is associated with prolonged transit, it has been postulated that constipation may show a monthly rhythm linked with the menstrual cycle. In controlled trials, however, such rhythmic patterns in constipation have not been found.

Does exercise improve bowel habits?

Mild exercise shortens whole gut transit time although stool weight and frequency of defaecation do not appear to be altered. Since daily exercise has such a wide range of added benefits, it can be profitably recommended to those wishing to improve their bowel habit.

Why are laxatives abused?

In addition to the misconceived belief that laxatives help in weight control, particularly after binge eating, some of those abusing laxatives report doing so to feel cleansed or empty and to 'flatten their tummies'.

Is high molecular weight polyethylene glycol effective as a laxative?

Polyethylene glycol 3350 is available as a powder formulation (Movicol) for the occasional treatment of chronic constipation. The powder also contains 178.5 mg sodium bicarbonate, 350.7 mg sodium chloride and 46.6 mg potassium chloride per sachet. This is equivalent to 65 mM Sodium, 5.4 mM of potassium, 53 mM of chloride and 17 mM of bicarbonate per sachet. Some limited data shows it to be effective in constipation but its place in relation to better established laxatives such as the sennosides has yet to be defined. For now, it should be regarded very much as a second-line agent and its salt content should be borne in mind when recommending it to patients.

Is hyoscine butylbromide effective in IBS?

Hyoscine butyl bromide is an antimuscarinic agent. It can therefore be expected to have some antispasmodic effects in IBS. As a quaternary ammonium compound it is poorly absorbed. This limits its efficacy as a gastro-intestinal antispasmodic.

What precautions should one observe with use of hyoscine butylbromide?

The limited extent to which the compound is absorbed also means that it is less likely to cause the well-known spectrum of systemic effects of hyoscine, namely confusion, dry mouth, glaucoma, hesitancy at micturation, constipation, problems with visual accommodation and even urinary retention in the elderly.

Precautions and when to refer

(R) If constipation alternates with diarrhoea (malignancy).

(R) If there is marked weight loss (malignancy).

(R) If associated with pain and bloating (more serious underlying pathology possible).

(R) If associated with thin pencil-like stools (irritable bowel syndrome).

(!) Be alert for possibility of laxative abuse.

(!) Take bulk laxatives with plenty of water.

(!) Do not take bulk laxatives immediately before going to bed.

(!) Dietary advice should always be given.

Selected product options

Irritable bowel syndrome

Colpermin EC Capsules
  (peppermint oil)
Fybogel mebeverine
  (mebeverine)

Mintec EC Capsules
  (peppermint oil)

Relaxyl Tablets (alverine
  citrate)

Constipation

Califig Syrup (sennosides)
Celevac Tablets (methylcellulose)
Duphalac Solution (lactulose)
Fybogel Granules (ispaghula husk)
Isogel Granules (ispaghula husk)

Regulan Granules (ispaghula husk)
Senlax Tablets (sennosides)
Senokot Granules (sennosides)
Senokot Syrup (sennosides)
Senokot Tablets (sennosides)

Second-line laxatives

Agarol Emulsion (phenolphthalein, liquid paraffin)
Alophen Pills (aloin, phenolphthalein)
Beechams Pills (aloin)
Bonomint Tablets (phenolphthalein)
Brooklax Tablets (phenolphthalein)
Carters Little Pills (aloin, phenolphthalein)
Dulco-lax Suppositories (bisacodyl)
Dulco-lax Tablets (bisacodyl)
Ex-Lax Tablets (phenolphthalein)
Ex-Lax Pills (phenolpohthalein)
Fleet Enema (sodium acid phosphate, sodium phosphate)
Fynnon Salt (sodium sulphate)
Herbulax Tablets (dandelion root, frangula dry extract)
Laxoberal Solution (sodium picosulphate)
Mil-Par Suspension (magnesium hydroxide)
Nylax Tablets (bisacodyl, phenolphthalein, senna leaf)
Potter's Cleaning Herb Tablets (senna leaves, aloes, cascara bark, dandelion root, fennel
  seed)
Regaletts Tablets (phenolphthalein)
Rhuaka Syrup (senna, cascara, rhubarb)
Sure-Lax Tablets (phenolphthalein)

Contact lenses

How many types of contact lenses are there and what are their relative merits?

There are now three broad categories of contact lenses:

- hard lenses
- soft lenses
- short-use disposable lenses.

The soft contact lenses may be designed for daily wear or alternatively for extended wear.

The hard lenses, often called hard gas-permeable lenses, provide excellent vision and are associated with very few eye infections. Initial fitting is more troublesome than with other types of lenses and adapting to them may take longer. On a longer term basis, they are easy to maintain and check. Cleaning and maintenance are straightforward and lens deposits and allergies are less likely. The backbone of hard lenses is typically made of silicone acrylates or fluoro-silicone acrylates. To improve lens comfort hydrophilic polymers such as N-vinyl pyrrolidone may be layered onto the acrylates. Fluorosilicones have higher oxygen permeabilities and fewer deposit problems than the silicone-based lenses. Reflections from the edges make the lenses more visible than soft lenses and their lower hydrophilicity makes them more likely to slide out and be lost.

Soft lenses are comfortable to wear from the initial fitting but quality of vision may be lower than is achievable with hard lenses. Soft lenses are retained on the eye better and are therefore better on the sports field. Oedema sometimes associated with hard lenses (particularly early on) is very rarely seen with soft lenses. However, scrupulous attention to regular lens disinfection is essential to avoid infection. Maintenance is expensive because of the greater propensity for a build-up of surface deposits and for damage. In principle, any lens which is well tolerated can be regarded as being biocompatible but more recently the descriptor has been given specifically to lenses made from materials such as phosphorylcholine used in transplant surgery.

Short-use disposable lenses include lenses which are replaced monthly or as frequently as daily. Build-up of surface deposits is overcome and the potential for eye infection induced by contaminated lenses essentially eliminated. Early suggestions that these lenses can be used for extended overnight wear are now regarded as unwise and patients should be advised to restrict wear to the waking hours.

What are the potential problems in the wearing of contact lenses?

Spoilage or spoilation of contact lenses, leading to intolerance to the lens, is often a problem, although in most cases the problem is transient. Intolerance may arise as a result of drying of the lens surface and subsequent denaturing of the proteins deposited. Heating of the lens without removal of the deposits causes further denaturation and the formation of more tenacious adsorbates. It is claimed that the intolerance may be immunological with the deposited proteins acting as antigens, or alternatively with the preservatives, present in contact lens solutions, acting as haptens. Atopic subjects appear to be more susceptible to intolerance to contact lenses thus providing some support for the immunological basis of the problem in at least some of the cases. In some instances, contact lenses are blamed for inducing dry eyes and most practitioners advise against the use of such lenses in those patients, although paradoxically some reports suggest that dry eyes may be successfully treated with soft contact lenses.

Spoilage of contact lenses may also be characterized by deposits other than of a proteinaceous nature. Calcium deposits, microbial deposits and iron deposition have been described. While the inorganic and proteinaceous deposits pose some problems by interfering with the clarity of the lenses and lead to lens intolerance, the most serious potential problem is the complex interaction between microbial deposits, lens surface and the corneal surface leading to infection. In this respect, fungal, pseudomonal, viral and amoebic infections are of particular concern.

In a recent study of 243 hydrophilic lenses, 100 were found to harbour fungi and pseudomonads could be cultured from 25 of them. Acanthamoebas, which are amoebas of trophozoites about $30l\mu m$ across, produce persistent keratitis and uveitis. Recently, the wearing of contact lenses has been identified as a serious risk factor to acanthamoebic infections.

Lens discoloration by ingested or applied drugs or their metabolites has also been reported and drugs implicated include adrenaline, rifampicin, amantadine and sulphasalazine. The adrenaline discoloration is thought to be due to adrenochrome or alternatively to melanin deposition enhanced by adrenaline.

What advice should contact lens wearers be given to avoid corneal infections?

The regular use of commercially available cleaning and wetting solutions should be encouraged and the use of saliva and home-made saline solutions as wetting and cleaning solutions should be strongly discouraged. Washing of hands prior to handling the lenses should be recommended. Visitors travelling to the tropics should be discouraged from wearing contact lenses because of the increased risk of acanthamoebic infections. Short-use disposable lenses are worthwhile replacements under such circumstances. Patients with dry eyes should be particularly careful in ensuring that the lenses do not dry out during use and atopic patients should avoid extended wear lenses. Where there is a previous history of sensitivity to eye drops or contact lens solutions, only sterile saline solutions should be used for cleaning or wetting of the lenses.

What types of lens are associated with a greater risk of corneal infections and who is most susceptible to such infections?

There appears to be a greater risk of infection with extended-wear contact lenses. Hard daily-wear lenses appear least likely to produce such infections. Elderly aphakic patients appear to be at greater risk than young myopic subjects. Atopic patients show more intolerance to contact lenses and may therefore be more susceptible to corneal infections when the lenses are worn. Patients on contraceptive pills are said to show more adverse reactions to contact lenses but this appears to be possibly true only for the older-type high ethinyloestradiol pills. Low-dose contraceptive pills do not appear to be associated with any increased risk of lens intolerance or lens-induced infections.

Precautions and when to refer_____

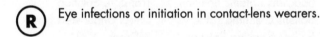 Eye infections or initiation in contact-lens wearers.

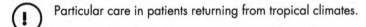 Particular care in patients returning from tropical climates.

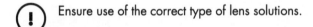 Ensure use of the correct type of lens solutions.

Product options _____

02 Care Solution
10:10 Cleaning and Disinfecting Solution
10:10 Rinsing and Neutralising Solution
10:10 System Five Pack
Adapettes Eye Drops
AMI-10 Solution
Amiclair Tablets
Amiclean Solution
Barnes-Hind Cleaner No. 4 Solution
Barnes-Hind Intensive Cleaner Solution
Barnes-Hind One Solution

Barnes-Hind Wetting and Soaking Solution
Barnes-Hind Wetting Solution
Bausch & Lomb Aerosol Saline Spray
Bausch & Lomb Daily Cleaner Solution
Boston Lens Wetting and Soaking Solution
Clean-N-Soak Solution
Clens Solution
Complete Care/Lensine Solution
Contactaclean Solution
Contactasoak Solution

Contactasol Solution
Flex-Care Solution
Flexsol Solution
Hexidin Solution
Hydrocare Cleaning/ Soaking Solution
Hydrocare Fizzy Tablet
Hydrocare Preserved Saline Solution
Hydrocare Protein Remover Tablets
Hydroclean Solution
Hydron Cleaning Solution
Hydron Comfort Solution

Hydron Saline BPH
Stabilised Sterile
Isotonic Saline Solution
Hydron Saline Pack
Tablets
Hydron Soaking Solution
Hydrosoak Solution
Hydrosol Solution
Kelsoak 2 Solution
Kelsoak Solution
Kelvinol 2 Solution
Kelvinol Solution
LC-65 Cleaning Solution
Lens Plus Spray
Lensept Solution
Lensept TE Opthalmic
Solution
Lensine 5 Solution
Lensrins Solution
Lensrins TE Buffered
Solution

Liquifilm Wetting Solution
Mediclean Solution
Medisoak Solution
Mira-Flow Solution
Mira-Soak Solution
Mira-Sol Solution
Normasol Solution
Normol Solution
Pliagel Solution
Preflex Solution
Prymecare Soluble Tablets
Prymeclean Solution
Prymesoak Solution
Salette Solution
Scanlens Rinse Solution
Septicon Disc
Snoflex Tablets
Soaclens Isotonic Solution
Soflens Cleaning Tablets
Soflens Soaking Solution
Softab Tablets

Solar Cleaning Solution
Solar Preserved Saline
Solution
Solar Saline Aerosol
Soquette Solution
Steri-Clens Solution
Steri-Fresh Eye Drops
Steri-Sal Solution
Steri-Solv Solution
TE Cleaning Solution
TE Storage and Rinsing
Solution
Titan Solution
Total Solution
Transclean Solution
Transoak Solution
Transol Solution
Transtore Solution
Unisol Unbuffered Eye
Drops

Contraceptive agents

What are the spermicidal compounds in current use?

Nonoxynol-9 is the most widely used spermicidal compound. Chlorhexidine and d-propranolol are currently being investigated and early results look promising. Benzalkonium compounds are already in use in France as spermicidal compounds.

How safe are vaginal spermicides?

One of the major concerns about the use of spermicides is whether failed spermicide contraception may lead to an increased lilkelihood of birth defects. Some early reports suggested some justification for that concern but subsequent reanalysis of the data indicated that after adjusting for maternal age, no association was found between spermicide failure and foetal abnormalities. A second concern relates to the toxicity of any absorbed spermicidal material. Much less is known about this risk although the amounts absorbed are likely to be small.

Are spermicidal sponges useful?

'Today' is a spermicide-impregnated polyurethane sponge currently available in the UK. The sponge may be worn for up to 30 hours but failure rates are relatively high.

Are films preferable to foams, gels or pessaries?

The choice really depends on the woman's preference. Films are regarded by some as being more elegant to use but they have to be inserted well before intercourse and may therefore be less acceptable. Foams are regarded as messy by some and stimulant by others. Used on its own, each spermicide is subject to a high failure rate relative to the condom and the contraceptive pill.

Do spermicides protect against sexually-transmitted diseases?

Nonoxynol-9 appears to protect against some sexually-transmitted diseases. However, only the condom appears to provide the necessary effectiveness against all such diseases, with proper use; hence the current campaign for the use of condoms against the spread of acquired immuno-deficiency syndrome (AIDS).

What are female condoms?

These are experimental condoms similar to the male condoms except that they are intended to be worn by the female partner and are of wider bore. Physically the female condom is a hybrid between the male condom and the diaphragm. Its acceptability, efficacy for preventing pregnancy and the spread of sexually transmitted diseases is as yet insufficiently tested.

How effective are condoms?

Used properly condoms should be 100% effective. However in use, tears and slippage may lead to failure and recent work on evaluating the properties of commercially available condoms revealed an alarming number of condoms with holes. The well-established brands tested to British Standards Institution specifications or other accepted standards should be recommended in preference to lesser known brands.

How effective are the diaphragms and caps?

The use of diaphragms is less popular than most alternative mainstream contraceptive methods. It is generally accepted that a second-line protection such as the concurrent use of a spermicidal foam is required whenever diaphragms are used as contraceptive devices. Excipients in some pessaries can interfere with the barrier function of diaphragms and whenever possible the rectal route should be used as an alternative to the vaginal route for delivering drugs whenever diaphragms are used as contraceptives.

What are post-coital methods of contraception?

Post-coital contraception, as the name suggests, is a method of preventing pregnancy after the sexual act. This method is usually applied up to 72 hours after unprotected intercourse. Douching is thought to be a post-coital contraception method by some but it is certainly an ineffective one. Early Egyptians are reported to have used garlic douches in this capacity. Current methods are based on the use of combination pills. The administration of two tablets each containing 50 mg of ethinyloestradiol and 250 mg levonorgestrel within 72 hours of unprotected intercourse and two more 12 hours later is a commonly used post-coital contraceptive regimen. Nausea and vomiting may be frequent side-effects but the incidence is low when compared with earlier methods which relied on diethylstilbestrol or ethinyloestradiol. Diethylstibestrol is now no longer used because of the link between its use and adenocarcinoma of the vagina in the adolescent female offspring. Copper intrauterine devices are also effective post-coital contraceptive devices and are recommended by some authorities particularly when the woman has decided to use an intrauterine contraceptive device (IUCD) for subsequent contraception.

More recently mefepristone (RU 486) has been introduced as a morning-after pill in a number of countries. However, although regulatory authorities such as the US Food and Drug Administration have recommended that mefepristone be approved, various lobbies such as the Pro-Life lobby in the USA are strongly opposed to this.

Does breast-feeding provide contraceptive cover?

Breast-feeding mothers resume menstruation later after parturition than do mothers who do not breast feed. In the presence of amenorrhoea and breast feeding, ovulation does not usually take place until after about the tenth post-partum week. However, it is estimated that up to 10% of women with lactational amenorrhoea become pregnant. In the presence of menstruation, an even higher proportion of breast-feeding mothers become pregnant. Therefore while breast feeding provides some contraceptive cover it is a highly unreliable method.

Which contraceptive method should then be recommended for nursing mothers?

The continuing uterine changes in the post-partum period make intrauterine devices (IUCDs) less suitable than alternative contraceptive methods. Pelvic inflammatory disease may also be more likely with IUCDs and barrier methods and steroidal contraceptive pills are more suitable alternatives. Any steroid secreted in breast milk appears to be of no consequence to the nursling. It also appears that the changes in the composition and volume of milk induced by oral contraceptives are small enough to be neglected. The progestogen only pill is usually recommended.

There has been much recent concern about the oral contraceptive pill. What are the main issues?

The most recent controversies have centred round an apparent increase in the risk of thrombotic events in users of the so-called 'third-generation' pills containing desogestrel or gestodene and an increased risk of breast cancer in women using oral contraceptives.

Several case-control studies have now consistently shown a small increased risk of venous thromboembolic events in users of desogestrel and gestodene-containing contraceptive pills. The UK Committee on Safety of Medicines were sufficiently concerned to advise restricting use of those agents to women who cannot tolerate other oestrogen–progestogen combination pills and to avoid their use in women at increased risk of thrombo-embolic events notably the obese and those with a previous history of such problems. Few other regulatory authorities however, concur with the CSM's view as the additional risk appears small.

A recent meta-analysis of case-control studies suggests that women who currently use or have recently used oral contraceptives have an increased risk of breast cancer. The odds ratio for current users relative to controls were 1.24 while for women who stopped using the pill one to four years earlier, the odds ratio was 1.16.

What is the toxic-shock syndrome?

This syndrome is a new disease which has been associated with the use of tampons during menstruation. However, the disease has also occurred in men and non-menstruating female patients, so tampons are not a sufficient or necessary cause. Typically the disease develops with sudden onset of fever, diarrhoea, shock, rashes, desquamation of hands and feet and hyperaemia of the hands, feet, vaginal mucous membranes and the oropharynx. Other organ systems may also be involved. The syndrome is commonly associated with the isolation of *Staphylococcus aureus* and the consensus view is that the disease is infective in origin. Most manufacturers have now withdrawn the highly absorbent tampons thought to be partly responsible for the syndrome and users are advised to change their tampons as regularly as possible. Barrier contraceptives are not implicated.

Are barrier methods safer than oral contraceptives?

Oral contraceptives are widely accepted to carry a potential to cause cardiovascular problems and a non-systemic method of contraception will clearly not carry this risk. Additionally, a recent study indicated that oral contraceptive and intrauterine device users show a shift in cervical flora from one in which Lactobacilli predominate to one in which anaerobic bacteria are the major component. However, there is no clear evidence that this shift has long-term health implications.

How do spermicides work?

The non-ionic spermicides appear to disrupt the lipid layer on the surface of the spermatozoa. Fructolytic metabolism is altered and sperm motility is impaired. The other agents in current use probably also exert their spermicidal activities through their surfactant properties.

Product options _____

(Products listed below appear safe for use with latex condoms and diaphragms)

Delfen Foam (nonoxynol-9)
Double Check Pessaries (nonoxynol-9)
Duracreme Cream (nonoxynol-9)
Duragel Gel (nonoxynol-9)

Gyno 11 (nonoxynol-9)
Ortho-Creme (nonoxynol-9)
Orthoforms Pessaries (nonoxynol-9)

Corns and calluses

What are corns and calluses?

Corns and calluses are hard keratinous areas of the skin caused by excessive localized pressure. Corns typically affect the feet as a result of the wearing of ill-fitting shoes while calluses affect both the feet and hands. Corns are also occasionally referred to as a localized tylosis or a heloma in the medical literature.

How should corns and calluses be treated?

Corns and calluses are best treated by removing the cause, namely the pressure caused by ill-fitting shoes or improper posture and excessive activity. Warm soaks followed by gentle rubbing with a pumice stone will help reduce the callosities. Use of a non-medicated corn pad may provide relief from pressure. For the isolated hard corn, a keratolytic corn pad will be useful. Emollient preparations may help improve the elasticity of the skin and provide symptomatic relief. Surgical removal by a chiropodist may be necessary for the persistent case. Great care must be exercised when treating diabetic patients and indeed, for such patients, self-treatment is not recommended.

Precautions and when to refer

(R) Refer diabetic patients.

(R) Patients with impaired peripheral vascular disturbance.

(R) Any bleeding lesion.

(!) Avoid eyes and mucous membranes.

Product options

Carnation Callous Pads (salicylic acid)
Freezone Liquid (salicylic acid)
Noxacorn (salicylic acid)
Scholl Callous Remover Plaster (salicylic acid)

Scholl Corn and Callous Removal Liquid (camphor, salicylic acid)
Scholl Corn Remover Plasters (salicylic acid)

Coughs

What causes coughing?

Coughing is a protective physiological reflex which clears the respiratory tract of both exogenous and endogenous irritants. The reflex is initiated by stimulation of cough receptors within the respiratory tract. The impulses are then passed along sensory nerves to the cough centre, a co-ordinating neuronal network in the brain medulla. Efferent impulses are then conveyed along cholinergic pathways to the diaphragm and the intercostal and abdominal muscles to produce the coughing action. Cough receptors are also located in other parts of the body including the ear and the stomach. Higher centres control the cough centre as is evident from the fact that the coughing reflex may be voluntarily initiated and suppressed, at least temporarily.

Should coughing be suppressed at all?

It can be argued that as a physiological protective mechanism, coughing should not be suppressed. However, in many instances coughing serves no useful function, being unproductive and exhausting. Under such circumstances, suppression of coughs is helpful to the patient. Productive coughs should not be suppressed and the use of antitussives should be avoided in the presence of increased sputum production as is observed in pertussis (whooping cough), chronic bronchitis and post-nasal drip.

How do cough suppressants work?

Cough suppressants may work by (a) blocking the cough receptors in the respiratory tract (demulcents and local anaesthetics), (b) depressing the cough centre (opiates, antihistamines and dextromethorphan) and (c) blockade at the motor nerves (local anaesthetics).

Which is the best antitussive agent?

Codeine phosphate is still the yardstick against which all the other antitussive agents are evaluated and there is little doubt that it is effective. However, its abuse potential and possible induction of respiratory depression are limitations which some authorities consider severe enough to warrant the drug's restriction to the prescription only medicine (POM) list. In the United Kingdom, cases of abuse have been reported to follow non-prescription use of codeine-containing cough linctuses. However, the problem seems to have been checked by voluntary monitoring of sales by pharmacists and careful supervision by the inspectorate of the pharmaceutical societies.

Dextromethorphan appears to be effective but less susceptible to abuse and induction of respiratory depression, though problems still surface on occasions and some regulatory authorities have reinitiated restriction of dextromethorphan on prescription sales. Pholcodine is an opiate derivative with a long half-life. It is not metabolized to morphine as has previously been erroneously claimed. Clinical trials to evaluate pholcodine's antitussive effects have yielded conflicting results. Noscapine is an opium alkaloid free from analgesic or narcotic activity. It is less likely than morphine or codeine to induce respiratory depression and constipation but the higher safety profile is unfortunately achieved at the expense of activity. Noscapine has until recently been available for sale as a general sales list (GSL) product but has now been withdrawn from sale in the United Kingdom as a result of suspected genotoxicity.

Diphenhydramine is an antihistamine which has been shown, in some studies, to be an active antitussive agent. Its effectiveness as a cough suppressant is probably due to its general central depressant activity. On this basis, the other sedative antihistamine (H$_1$) compounds probably share the antitussive activity of diphenhydramine.

Which is the best antitussive for infants?

Many authorities are of the opinion that coughing should not normally be suppressed in infants except under extreme circumstances. Indeed none of the standard antitussives are recommended for OTC use in infants because of possible respiratory depression, particularly with codeine. The use of the antitussives needs careful consideration in the presence of chronic pulmonary disease and shortness of breath in all age groups, but in particular in infants. In older children whenever codeine is used, careful dosing is required.

Are expectorants useful?

Mucus secretion forms part of the defensive or protective mechanisms operating in the respiratory tract and increased secretion during microbial attack of the respiratory tract is therefore to be expected. Often, however, the secretions become tenacious, impede breathing and cause discomfort. Under these circumstances, an expectorant appears worthwhile. However, none of the available expectorants appears to be any more effective than simple linctuses. Ipecacuanha, ammonium chloride and terpin hydrate, at expectorant doses, are probably no more than mere placebos. Guaiphenesin, also known as glyceryl guaicolate and guaicol glycerol, at a 100 mg dose is widely held to be effective but the supporting evidence is limited. Steam inhalations are effective expectorants but their use requires much motivation.

All the commonly used expectorants are generally safe at the dosages usually recommended. Iodides were previously widely used but their potential adverse effects on the thyroid gland has led to their gradual phasing out from expectorant formulations. Painful swelling of the salivary and lacrimal glands, unpleasant metallic tastes, heartburn, nausea and vomiting are other potential adverse effects. Iodides should also be avoided during pregnancy and lactation because of possible toxicity, in particular on the thyroid gland, in the foetus and newborn.

Are inhalations and menthol-containing ointments useful for the control of coughing?

Steam inhalations may be helpful in loosening phlegm and indeed despite some contradictory evidence the FDA considers menthol (0.05%) and camphor (0.1%) inhalations effective and safe for the relief of coughs. Ointments containing 4.7 to 5.3% camphor or 2.6 to 2.8% menthol are also considered effective by the same agency, for the relief of coughs when applied to the throat or chest. Such ointments are contraindicated for intranasal use and should not be used in infants as toxic reactions have been reported following the use of camphor-containing products in the young. Some recent data suggest that menthol may act as a calcium channel blocker and hence vasodilator.

Are mucolytic agents useful expectorants?

Mucolytics break down mucus to produce a less viscous fluid which should theoretically be easier to expectorate. However, there is insufficient evidence of their effectiveness to justify their recommendation.

Which cough product can be recommended for diabetics?

A number of sugar-free cough mixtures are now available based on sorbitol, lycasin and their mixtures with saccharin. The lycasin-based formulations, being metabolized to glucose, are not recommended. Sorbitol and saccharin-based formulations are suitable alternatives to sucrose-based formulations for the diabetic although their advantages are often over-emphasized.

Some drugs are reported to induce coughing. How do they cause this?

A number of drugs including pentamidine, busulphan and angiotensin-converting enzyme (ACE) inhibitors have been reported to induce cough. Indeed some reports suggest that some ACE inhibitors may cause coughing in as many as 10% of patients. The mechanism of action is unclear although ACE inhibitors are known to impair ciliary beat in the trachea.

Precautions and when to refer

(R) If wheeziness present.

(R) Whooping cough.

(R) Recurrent nocturnal coughing.

(R) Persistent coughing (> 3 weeks).

(R) Cough with chest pain or pus-loaded or bloody sputum.

(R) Cough with shortness of breath.

(!) Cough may be drug-induced. Pay particular attention to ACE inhibitors, busulphan and pentamidine.

(!) Avoid theophylline in acute porphyria.

(!) Avoid dextromethorphan in children with a history of CNS problems.

(!) Avoid codeine and dextromethorphan in patients with a history of drug abuse.

(!) Avoid paediatric formulations containing decongestants, particularly late at night.

Product options

For dry coughs
Actifed Junior Cough Relief (dextromethorphan, triprolidine)
Benylin Children's Coughs (diphenhydramine)
Benylin Children's Coughs Sugar Free (diphenhydramine)
Benylin Dry Coughs Non-Drowsy (dextromethorphan)
Benylin Dry Coughs Original (dextromethorphan, diphenhydramine)
Benylin with Codeine (codeine, diphenhydramine)
Bronalin Junior Linctus (diphenhydramine)
Buttercup Syrup (squill extract, capsicum)
Contac Cough Caps (dextromethorphan)
Covonia Bronchial Balsam (dextromethorphan)
Covonia for Children Linctus (dextromethorphan)

Expulin Dry Cough Linctus (pholcodine)
Famel Linctus (pholcodine)
Franolyn Dry Cough (dextromethorphan)
Hill's Balsam Adult Suppressant Mixture (pholcodine)
Lemsip Dry Tickly Cough Linctus (honey, glycerin)
Meltus Baby Linctus (no actives)
Meltus Cough Control Capsules (dextromethorphan)
Nirolex Lozenges (dextromethorphan)
Owbridge's Children's Cough Mixture (diphenhydramine)
Owbridge's For Dry Coughs (dextromethorphan)
Pavacol – D Syrup (pholcodine)
Robitussin Dry Cough (dextromethorphan)
Robitussin Junior Persistent Cough Medicine (dextromethorphan)
Terpoin Syrup (codeine phosphate)
Tixylix Daytime Linctus (pholcodine)
Tixylix Nightime Linctus (promethazine, pholcodine)
Veno's Cough Mixture (no actives)
Veno's Honey and Lemon Syrup
Vicks Original Cough Syrup, Dry, Tickly (no actives)
Vicks Vaposyrup for Dry Coughs Syrup (dextromethorphan)

Expectorants
Benylin Chesty Coughs, Non-Drowsy (guaiphenesin)
Boots Children's Chesty Cough Syrup (guaiphenesin)
Buttercup Blackcurrant Syrup (ipecacuanha)
Dodo Expectorant Linctus (guaiphenesin)
Galloways Cough Syrup (ipecacuanha, squill)
Hill's Expectorant (guaiphenesin)
Hill's Balsam Children's Mixture for Chesty Coughs (ipecacuanha)
Hill's Balsam Pastilles for Chesty Coughs (ipecacuanha)
Jackson's All Fours Syrup (guaiphenesin)
Lemsip Chesty Cough Linctus (guaiphenesin)
Liquifruta Cough Medicine (ipecacuanha)
Liquifruta Garlic Cough Medicine (guaiphenesin)
Meltus Adult Expectorant Linctus (guaiphenesin)
Meltus Cough Linctus Honey and Lemon (guaiphenesin)
Meltus Junior Expectorant Linctus (guaiphenesin)
Nurse Sykes Balsam (guaiphenesin)
Owbridge's for Chesty Coughs (guaiphenesin)
Tixylix Chesty Cough Linctus (guaiphenesin)
Veno's Expectorant (guaiphenesin)
Vicks Original Syrup, Chesty (guaiphenesin)
Vicks Vaposyrup for Chesty Coughs (guaiphenesin)

Decongestant cough products
Actifed Expectorant (guaiphenesin, pseudoephedrine)
Dimotane Expectorant (guaiphenesin, pseudoephedrine)
Dodo Chesteze (ephedrine, theophylline)
Franolyn Chesty Coughs (guaiphenesin, theophylline, ephedrine)
Nirolex (guaiphenesin, ephedrine)
Robitussin Chesty Cough with Congestion (guaiphenesin, pseudoephedrine)
Vicks Vaposyrup for Chesty Coughs and Nasal Congestion (guaiphenesin, phenylpropanolamine)

Products with seemingly irrational combinations or mislabelled

Actifed Compound Linctus (dextromethorphan, pseudoephedrine)
Adult Meltus for Dry Tickly Coughs and Catarrh (dextromethorphan, pseudoephedrine)
Benylin Cough and Congestion (dextromethorphan, pseudoephedrine)
Bronalin Dry Cough Elixir (dextromethorphan, pseudoephedrine)
Dimotane Co Liquid (codeine, pseudoephedrine)
Dimotane Co Paediatric (codeine, pseudoephedrine, brompheniramine)
Ecdylin Syrup (ammonium chloride, diphenhydramine)
Expulin Cough Linctus (chorpheniramine, pseudoephedrine, pholcodine)
Histalix Syrup (ammonium chloride, diphenhydramine)
Meltus Junior Dry Cough Elixir (dextromethorphan, pseudoephedrine)
Pulmo Bailly (guaiacol, codeine)
Sudafed Linctus (dextromethorphan, pseudoephedrine)
Vicks Vaposyrup for Dry Cough and Nasal Congestion Syrup (dextromethorphan, phenylpropanolamine)

Paediatric formulations with decongestants

Dimotapp Co Paediatric (codeine, pseudoephedrine)
Secron Syrup for Children (ephedrine)

Cystitis

What is cystitis?

Cystitis refers to inflammation of the bladder but clinically cystitis defines a syndrome characterized by urinary urgency, pain on micturation and constant urge to pass water to alleviate the irritation.

What causes cystitis?

In about half of the cases, cystitis is caused by microbial infection of the urinary tract. In the other cases no micro-organism can be isolated although as yet unidentified infective agents could well be involved.

Which are the commonest infective organisms in cystitis?

E. coli is the commonest, thus suggesting a possible faecal source of contamination. Proteus species are also common isolates.

What is the best therapy for cystitis?

Specific antimicrobial chemotherapy is clearly the most logical approach when the causative micro-organism can be isolated and tested for sensitivity to antimicrobial agents. For many patients repeated microbial cultures yield negative results and no underlying pathology can be identified. For these patients symptomatic treatment with non-specific agents is suitable.

How useful are urinary alkalinizing agents?

Urine alkalinizing agents such as bicarbonates, antacids and citric acid salts are widely used and many sufferers find them useful for relieving the discomfort associated with cystitis. However, indiscriminate use is not justified since only in *E. coli* infections is the urine acidic. With proteus infections the urine is in fact alkaline and alkalinizing agents will clearly be illogical for treating those cases. For the remaining half of the cases alkalinizing agents are likely to be no better than increased fluid intake. The latter should perhaps be the treatment of first choice when symptomatic relief of cystitis is required. Counter prescribing barley water, chicken essence or mineral water is likely to be as logical as counterprescribing potassium or sodium citrate mixtures.

Is it true that women are more common cystitis sufferers than men?

This is indeed the case except in the elderly when the relative incidence in the two sexes is reversed. Prostate gland enlargement is the major reason for the increasing incidence of cystitis in elderly males. Females suffer more often from cystitis than males possibly because of the shorter urethra in the female than in the male.

What are the other predisposing factors to cystitis?

Physical abrasion to the outer urinary tract is a predisposing factor to cystitis as is chemical irritation. Cases labelled as 'honeymoon' cystitis and 'bubble bath' cystitis have been described in the literature. In fact certain female cystitis sufferers are prescribed prophylactic doses of antimicrobial agents to pre-empt cystitis attacks after sexual intercourse. Voiding of the bladder immediately after intercourse is also often recommended to these sufferers. Any condition or drug which interferes with efficient voiding of the bladder will also predispose to cystitis. Prostate gland enlargement and anticholinergic drugs are two examples. Use of the diaphragm has also been associated with an increased incidence of cystitis.

Is cystitis dangerous?

Fortunately most cases of cystitis are self-limiting and produce no lasting damage to the urinary tract. Only when the cystitis is secondary to a more serious pathological condition or when the upper urinary tract is involved is there cause for alarm.

When should a more serious pathology than primary cystitis be suspected?

Haematuria or blood in urine is always a cause for concern. Cytotoxic therapy and schistosomiasis or bilharzia are two possible causes of secondary cystitis presenting with haematuria.

How does methenamine or hexamine work?

Methenamine is a prodrug of formaldehyde and is therefore essentially an anti-microbial agent. The formaldehyde is only released in the presence of an acidic urine and concurrent use with large regular doses of antacids or with sodium or potassium citrate is therefore contraindicated.

Why has methenamine been withdrawn by some manufacturers?

The reasons for the withdrawal of pharmaceutical products from the market-place by manufacturers are often complex. Low sales volume and the potential toxicity of formaldehyde are no doubt contributory factors to the withdrawal of methenamine-containing products in the UK. Lack of efficacy does not appear to be a problem with methenamine and some literature in fact suggests that resistance to it is less likely than to conventional antimicrobial agents.

Is phenazopyridine hydrochloride effective in cystitis?

Phenazopyridine hydrochloride is used for the relief of pain associated with cystitis. As a palliative it is less safe than the citrates, as indicated by the reports of liver dysfunction following its use. Calculi formation has also been reported. There is therefore little justification for the continued use of phenazopyridine hydrochloride.

Is cranberry juice useful in cystitis?

Cranberry juice has for decades been thought to be useful in cystitis. It was originally thought that the juice acidified urine thereby exerting a bacteriostatic effect. However recent studies suggest that the juice did not necessarily lower urinary pH and a more likely mechanism might be inhibition of bacterial adherence to uroepithelial cells. Irrespective of the putative mechanism of action, it was not until very recently that a well controlled trial of the effect of ingestion of the juice on preventing cystitis was undertaken. Elderly women randomized to consuming 300 ml of cranberry juice per day were less likely to suffer from bacteriuria with pyuria than were control subjects receiving placebo with the same vitamin C content. Whether cranberry juice is effective in active cystitis is not yet known but clearly the rationale for recommending the juice appears sound.

Is saw palmetto useful in cystitis?

Products containing saw palmetto fruits are widely used in Germany for the symptomatic treatment of benign prostate hyperplasia. There is no good clinical trial evidence to show that it is better than placebo in this condition or in cystitis.

Precautions and when to refer

(R) Patients with fever or vomiting.

(R) Males with cystitis (prostate enlargement).

(R) Children with cystitis (general precaution and child abuse).

(R) Patients with loin or back pain.

(R) Patients with persistent cystitis (> 3 days).

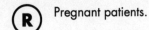 Pregnant patients.

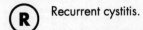 Recurrent cystitis.

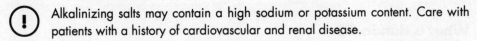 Alkalinizing salts may contain a high sodium or potassium content. Care with patients with a history of cardiovascular and renal disease.

Avoid use of Effercitrate, potassium citrate mixture and other potassium-containing alkalinizers with ACE inhibitors, cyclosporin, spironolactone, amiloride, triamterene and potassium canrenoate because of increased risk of hyperkalaemia.

Product options

Cymalon Granules
(sodium citrate)

Cystoleve Powders
(sodium citrate)

Cystopurin Powders
(potassium citrate)

Dandruff

What is dandruff?

Dandruff is a condition characterized by excessive shedding of the cornified cells of the scalp, in the form of flakes or squames.

What causes dandruff?

A clear answer to this problem is still not available. It is known that dandruff is accompanied by an increased epidermal turnover and that antimicrobial agents are effective in controlling dandruff. However, it is not possible to determine whether the micro-organisms are aetiological or whether they are secondary to an increased epidermal cell turnover. An increasing number of experts, however, now favour the microbial aetiology of dandruff.

Which organisms are most often associated with dandruff?

Three types of organisms can readily be isolated from the scalp whether acne is present or not. These are the yeast *Pytyrosporum ovale*, the gram positive rod *Propionobacterium acnes* and the aerobic cocci. *P. ovale*. The yeast appears to be the organism most commonly associated with dandruff.

What types of remedies are available for the treatment of dandruff?

The remedies commonly used for the control of dandruff include (1) topical corticosteroids, (2) topical antimicrobial agents, (3) selenium sulphide, (4) zinc pyrithione, (5) tar extracts and (6) keratolytic agents.

How do selenium sulphide, zinc pyrithione and tar extracts exert their anti-dandruff activities?

All three are commonly thought to exert their anti-dandruff activities through a cytostatic or antimitotic activity. However, a number of authors have produced data to show that zinc pyrithione probably owes its activity more to its inhibitory effect on *p. Ovale* than to any cytostatic activity which it may have.

What are the best treatments available for dandruff?

The available treatments for dandruff may be classified into one of four groups: (1) corticosteroids for topical application, (2) antimicrobial products, (3) keratolytic formulation and (4) tar products.

Corticosteroidal products are prescribed by a number of practitioners but generally only when treatment with keratolytic or antimicrobial formulations has failed. This restriction is clearly rational and to be encouraged.

Keratolytic formulations are not cosmetically pleasant or easy to apply to hairy areas and therefore are not the treatment of choice for dandruff. Keratolytic shampoos do not allow sufficient contact time for truly effective action beyond that provided by the surfactant base alone.

The most rational approach to dandruff therefore appears to be the regular use of a suitable antimicrobial shampoo. Although a wide array of such shampoos are available, three classes stand out in terms of effectiveness, namely those containing zinc pyrithione, selenium sulphide, and ketoconazole.

Zinc pyrithione is available in the form of pleasant shampoos at relatively low prices. Among the commercially most successful formulations are Head and Shoulders and All Clear. Although zinc pyrithione shampoos are effective in controlling dandruff, regular use is required. They are also claimed to increase the greasiness of hair. Generic or own-brand formulations appear to be as effective as the brand leaders.

What advice should be given to patients using the anti-dandruff formulations?

More frequent shampooing at the start of therapy is required. Regular use of the anti-dandruff agents, most notably of selenium sulphide, ketoconazole and zinc pyrithione, is necessary to prevent relapse.

Is it true that selenium sulphide may cause hair loss?

Hair loss following use of selenium sulphide has been reported but this has not been confirmed by subsequent work.

Precautions and when to refer

Cases which do not respond to regular use of zinc pyrithione shampoo.

Product options

Lenium Shampoo (selenium sulphide)
Nizoral Shampoo (ketoconazole)

Selsun Shampoo (selenium sulphide)
Any shampoo containing zinc pyrithione.

Deodorants

Does increased perspiration lead to body odour?

Fresh sweat is usually odourless although admixture with apocrine secretions may give it an odour which may be partly genetically determined. Unpleasant body odours are generally associated with microbiologically decomposed components of the sweat and more particularly of apocrine secretions, although a number of clinical conditions (Table 10) may be associated with such odours. As is obvious from Table 10, body odours are not always cutaneous in origin.

Table 10 Sources of body odour.

Source	Possible basis
Imaginary	Psychiatric
Breath	Diabetes, ingested food metabolites
	Vincent's angina
	Nasal and URT infections or carcinoma
	Lung abscesses, bronchiectasis
Cutaneous	Topical applications (cosmetics, medicinal)
	Hidradenitis suppuritiva
	Ulcerated wounds
	Infections
	Fournier's gangrene
	Darier's disease
	Malignancy
	Stale sebum and sweat
	Food metabolites (garlic)
	Metabolites arising from inherited metabolic disorders (e.g. phenylketonuria, hypermethionienaemia, isovaleric acidaemia, trimethylamineuria)
Urinary	Incontinence
	Proteus vulgaris infections
Rectal	Soiling
	Haemorrhoids, fissures
Vaginal	Infections, menstrual exudates

Which are the most effective deodorant formulations?

While perfumes are sometimes useful masking agents for body odours, the most effective deodorant formulations usually include an effective antiseptic compound to inhibit the growth of micro-organisms responsible for breaking down apocrine gland secretions to malodorous compounds. Chlorhexidine is widely used in this respect.

Are deodorant powders safe to use?

Deodorant powders are usually formulated from antiseptics and perfumes absorbed on a chemically inert earth such as talc. Two types of worries have been raised in the literature. The first concerns toxicity of the antiseptic components and the perfumes and the second relates to absorption of the inert earths through the lungs or the vagina. The most widely publicized toxic reactions to the antiseptic components of topically applied powders have involved hexachlorophane and boric acid. Many of the more serious reactions have followed the use of incorrectly formulated powders. Nonetheless, the adverse publicity has led to stringent regulatory controls in the use of these two antiseptics and reports of their toxicity are now exceedingly rare. There has also been a gradual shift to the use of safer compounds such as chlorhexidine and triclosan (Irgasan DP300). Bithionol is now no longer recommended because of its potential phototoxicity.

Inhalation of particles of talc or of other commonly used powders are generally thought to be non-hazardous unless contaminated by asbestos particles. The quality control of the inert powders are now stringent to ensure freedom from such particles. Intra-vaginal contamination by talcum powder is also unlikely to lead to clinical problems.

Are antiperspirant aerosols safe?

Antiperspirant aerosols may be formulated as dry aerosols or as aerosol suspensions. Dry aerosols may contain an inert carrier, in which case the potential problems are as discussed for deodorant powders. An additional problem is linked with the formation of axillary granulomata, particularly when the fine aerosols are directed at shaven armpits or at abraded or irritated skin. Both the active antiperspirant compound and the inert powder carrier may cause the granulomata and both aluminium and zirconium salts have been implicated.

How does aluminium chloride work as an antiperspirant?

The mode of action of aluminium chloride as an antiperspirant is still unclear despite extensive use of the compound. Current data, however, suggest that the site of activity of the aluminium salt is not the secretory gland but is most likely to be the sweat duct. Suggestions put forward include plugging of the ducts by aluminium hydroxide formed on neutralization of the chloride and increased permeability of the epidermal portion of the duct leading to sweat resorption.

When should excessive sweating be investigated?

Excessive sweating should be investigated whenever there is no obvious cause. Hot flushes and sweating are often part of the menopausal syndrome. Diabetes may be associated with marked nocturnal sweating as may hepatic pathology. Hodgkin's lymphoma may present with sweating as a major symptom although weight loss, weakness and marked adenopathy are more characteristic features. Among new immigrants from countries where tuberculosis is endemic, nocturnal sweating may be a symptom of tuberculosis. Malaria is of course characterized by regular bouts of fever and sweating and the infection should be excluded in feverish patients returning from malarious areas. Sometimes sweating is purely psychogenic and treatment of associated anxiety states is required.

Precautions and when to refer_____

Patients with unexplained body odour.

Diarrhoea

What is diarrhoea?

The readily perceptible features of diarrhoea are known to all. Even children are quite able to diagnose diarrhoea by themselves. Biochemically, diarrhoea is a disturbance in intestinal electrolyte and water transport. Under normal circumstances the intestinal epithelium is able to maintain balance between secretion and absorption. The villous epithelium absorbs water and sodium ions while the crypt epithelium secretes water and chloride ions. Both of these processes are under the influence of neuroendocrine transmitters, hormones and other intestinal substances.

In the presence of toxic stimuli arising from enterotoxins, infection or cellular damage by infections, homeostasis is disturbed and diarrhoea follows. With severe diarrhoea such as that associated with cholera, as much as 20 litres of water may be lost per 24 hours. Diarrhoea may also be induced by an alteration in intestinal transport and by an accumulation of osmotically-active agents in the intestinal lumen.

How do anti-diarrhoeal agents work?

Anti-diarrhoeal agents may exert beneficial effects via three distinct mechanisms: (1) antimicrobial activity against any offending micro-organisms, (2) stimulation of absorption of water and electrolytes and (3) decreasing stimulated water and anion secretion. A fourth mechanism, put forward to claim activity for agents such as kaolin and attapulgite, is that of physical adsorption and inactivation of toxins and microbes. There is conflicting evidence about the likelihood of this mechanism operating successfully in the *in-vivo* situation.

Intuitively one would expect administration of electrolyte solution to make diarrhoea worse. Why do rehydration solutions help?

Indeed, this intuitive expectation is so strong that in the past, withholding fluids was one form of anti-diarrhoeal therapy which was applied with disastrous consequences. In some communities, it is still difficult to persuade parents that additional fluids and electrolytes are all that are required for most cases of diarrhoea. Rehydration fluids produce a beneficial effect in diarrhoea by increasing water absorption via the sodium absorption process.

In severe acute diarrhoea, rehydration fluid is the treatment of choice. In most cases of diarrhoea, in otherwise healthy adults, the fluid and electrolyte loss is small enough to be adequately managed by an increased fluid intake (water, soups, fruit juices). Electrolyte imbalance may be rapidly induced in the very young and the elderly. Particular care is therefore required in managing such patients.

What causes traveller's diarrhoea?

In the past, traveller's diarrhoea was often attributed to 'constitutional' upset. It is now known that most cases are attributable to infection by pathogenic strains of *Escherichia coli*. Non-pathogenic strains are permanent residents of the large intestine. Although these non-pathogenic strains are found at a density of about 10^5 to 10^8 cells per gram of faecal material, they only represent a tiny proportion of the total bacterial density of faecal material which is of the order of 10^{11} cells/g.

The pathogenic strains of *E. coli* can be identified by their ability to produce enterotoxins and/or to attach themselves to the intestinal wall and to invade the epithelial cells. Salmonella, campylobacter and giardia may cause persistent diarrhoea in travellers returning from Mediterranean and tropical countries. Amoebic dysentery caused by the protozoa *Entamoeba histolytica* may cause bloody diarrhoea. *Cryptosporidium parvum*, another protozoa, is also being increasingly recognized as a cause of diarrhoea in men.

What are the causes of food poisoning?

Pathogenic *Escherichia coli* infections of the gastrointestinal tract may be regarded as a form of food poisoning. However, more commonly the term food poisoning is ascribed to outbreaks caused by salmonella, campylobacter and clostridium species. Such outbreaks are often associated with closed communities such as hospital wards and old-people's homes. The increased consumption of contaminated fresh chickens and liquid egg-products is thought to have contributed to recent rises in the incidence of food poisoning. *Clostridium botulism* is a relatively rare cause of food poisoning but its toxin may be deadly. Occasional deaths are reported, particularly in relation to inadequately processed tinned foods such as corned beef and salmon. *Clostridium welchii* is the more common species involved in food poisoning in this country. Fortunately it is also much less dangerous. Colicky abdominal pain and diarrhoea are characteristic symptoms.

A different type of food poisoning is associated with ingestion of shell-fish and poorly-stored fish. With shell-fish, toxins produced by dinoflagellate protozoa are thought responsible, while with fish such as mackerel, tuna and sardines, a toxin referred to as a scombrotoxin is thought to be involved. Gastro-intestinal symptoms, including diarrhoea, are relatively mild but are accompanied by other disturbances such as muscle weakness, nausea and vomiting. With the dinoflagellates, neurotoxins may cause paralysis and death in some cases. Food poisoning may therefore be caused by a variety of micro-organisms and toxins and symptoms range from mild diarrhoea to potentially lethal disturbances.

Food poisoning not characterized by diarrhoea may also be seen. An example which has caused much recent concern is Listeriosis. The infection caused by the bacterium *Listeria monocytogenes* is particularly dangerous to the foetus, with abortions and still-births being common sequels. Cheeses made with non-pasteurized milk and cook–chill foods are particularly common sources of the bacterium.

Should milk be avoided during and immediately after diarrhoeal attacks?

Avoidance of milk was indeed, at one time, standard advice in the management of diarrhoea based on the recognition that lactase deficiency was a common complication of diarrhoeal attacks. Lactose intolerance could be identified after gastro-enteritis, in over half of the patients, until about the middle seventies. Over the past decade, lactose intolerance has become an increasingly rare complication of diar-rhoea among infants. This trend is not fully explained but it has been suggested that the modern adapted milk formulae present a milder challenge to the intestines than did the earlier high–solute formulae. Therefore the challenge rather than the pathological changes appear to have undergone the beneficial transformation leading to a lower incidence of lactose intolerance. On current evidence there is little justification for withholding milk-feeds based on breast-milk or on standard adapted milk-formulae in diarrhoea. Withholding unmodified cow's milk is still sound advice both for the young and for adults.

Are lactobacillus and yoghurt-based products useful in diarrhoea?

There is no convincing evidence that they are. However, yoghurt would be an acceptable food during diarrhoea since lactose, normally present in milk, is fully hydrolysed in yoghurt. Therefore, even in the presence of gastroenteritis-induced lactose intolerance, yoghurt is acceptable.

How does codeine control diarrhoea?

Codeine and opiates in general work by altering water and electrolyte transport and by reducing intestinal motility, particularly jejunal motor activity. Codeine appears to act on μ opiate receptors in the gut. The net result is a decrease in stool water.

How does loperamide work?

Loperamide is structurally related to the opiates but is essentially free of their narcotic activities. The drug binds to μ opiate receptors much like codeine and in healthy volunteers the drug decreases intestinal motor activity. The drug also inhibits prostaglandin E_2-induced secretion of water, sodium, potassium and chloride. Rectal sphincter-tone is also increased by the drug, a feature which makes it useful in faecal incontinence. Stimulation of δ opiate receptors which mediate basal water and electrolyte absorption has also been claimed for loperamide but the evidence is still inconclusive.

Should loperamide be used in preference to the classical opiates?

There is unfortunately little published work comparing the anti-diarrhoeal activities of codeine, morphine and loperamide. At non-prescription doses, formulations currently available in the United Kingdom are unpalatable enough or weak enough to present little risk of addictions. Lack of good published reports suggests that the formulations are probably not as potent as the marketing people would have us believe. The same applies to loperamide, although on the whole the evidence seems to be better for loperamide than for the non-prescription standard codeine or morphine-containing formulations. The essentially non-narcotic nature of loperamide is of course a major advantage. However, some regulatory authorities have yet to be convinced that loperamide, codeine and morphine are safe or effective enough for non-prescription use. Loperamide has been associated with severe adverse reactions in overdose.

Is there still a place for Kaolin and Morphine Mixture for the treatment of diarrhoea?

Research on the anti-diarrhoeal activities of the mixture has failed to show any positive results. The formulation has served us well in the past as a useful placebo in the treatment of diarrhoea. Most of the perceived effectiveness of anti-diarrhoeal agents used on a self-treatment basis is probably due to a placebo effect. In this sense, Kaolin and Morphine Mixture remains a worthwhile alternative to the more modern formulations, but many authorities disapprove.

How is bismuth subsalicylate thought to work in the control of diarrhoea?

Bismuth subsalicylate suspension is a relatively recent introduction for the treatment of diarrhoea and published results suggests that it is useful for the prevention and treatment of traveller's diarrhoea. Its mode of action is complex. The drug hydrolyses to bismuth and salicylic acid. The latter is of course well known for its anti-prostaglandin synthetase activity. Hence an inhibitory effect on intestinal secretion can be expected from ingestion of bismuth subsalicylate. A direct effect of bismuth on enterotoxigenic *E. coli*, the organism most commonly associated with traveller's diarrhoea, has also been suggested. Bismuth salicylate may be absorbed systemically and is not recommended as a first-line therapy for diarrhoea. The product has now been voluntarily withdrawn from sale by the manufacturers in the United Kingdom.

Can new and more effective anti-diarrhoeal agents be expected?

Progress in this field has been painfully slow but major advances have been made over the past decade and novel anti-diarrhoeal agents are likely to stem from those recent discoveries. Agents currently under investigation include, (1) α_2 agonists such as clonidine and lidamidine, (2) somatostatin, an inhibitor of intestinal motility although paradoxically diarrhoea often seems to be associated with a decrease in intestinal motility, (3) prostaglandins which modulate water transport, (4) calcium and calmodulin antagonists such as verapamil and phenothiazines because of their effects in decreasing intraluminal water accumulation, (5) enkephalins which increase basal sodium and chloride absorption, (6) berberine, a naturally-occurring alkaloid and (7) nicotinic acid. A thorough evaluation of their effectiveness in diarrhoea is likely to take at least a few more years.

Can drug therapy be a cause of diarrhoea?

A number of drugs may indeed induce diarrhoea as an adverse effect. Surreptitious laxative abuse and excessive intakes of vitamin E and sorbitol-containing confectionery may be associated with diarrhoea as may drug therapy with broad-spectrum antibiotics, guanethidine, methyldopa, digoxin, quinidine, chloroquine and anti-cancer drugs.

Is it possible to use oral vaccines against the diarrhoea-causing agents?

In theory it should be possible to obtain an effective vaccine against travellers' diarrhoea but the wide range of organisms involved makes the realization of such a vaccine difficult. However, in one recent study, administration of an oral buffered bovine milk immunoglobulin raised against the majority of *Escherichia coli*, known to be enterotoxigenic, led to protection against these organisms. The *E. coli* were administered 15 minutes prior to a dose of the immunoglobulin product which was also additionally given three times daily. Whether this approach is effective in the field situation remains to be determined. Lactobacilli are on the whole disappointing as anti-diarrhoeal prophylactic agents.

Precautions and when to refer

(R) Diarrhoea in the young, elderly and the pregnant.

(R) Diarrhoea with fever, traces of blood or vomiting.

(R) Diarrhoea acquired in Mediterranean or tropical countries.

(R) Chronic diarrhoea or diarrhoea alternating with constipation.

(R) Diarrhoea accompanying or following antibiotic therapy.

(R) Diarrhoea in the apparently anorexic patient.

Avoid use of loperamide in children.

 Avoid use of antispasmodics in children.

Product options

Rehydration fluids
Diocalm Replenish Powder   Dioralyte Powder   Glucolyte Powder
Dioralyte Tablets

Antidiarrhoeal agents
Diocalm Ultra Capsules (loperamide)   J Collis Browne's Tablets (morphine)
Imodium Capsules (loperamide)   Kaodene Suspension (codeine)
J Collis Browne's Mixture (morphine)

Placebo mixtures (?)
Kaopectate Suspension (kaolin)   KLN Suspension (kaolin)

Dry eye

What is the dry eye syndrome?

The dry eye syndrome or keratoconjunctivitis sicca, is characterized by a feeling of grit in the eye, heaviness of the lids, difficulty in opening the eyes and occasionally headache. The disease is often associated with old age. There may also be an association with dry mouth in Sjögren's syndrome.

What causes dry eye (keratoconjunctivitis sicca)?

The normal adult tear film which is about 10µ thick consists of three distinct layers: a mucus layer next to the epithelium, an intermediate aqueous layer and a superficial lipid layer secreted by the meibomian glands of the eyes. Dry eye is caused by inadequate secretion by (1) the mucus-secreting globet cells, (2) the lacrimal glands or (3) the meibomian glands, leading to instability and break-down of the tear film. The inadequate secretion may be part of the ageing process or more rarely may be due to ingested drugs such as anticholinergic agents or the beta blockers.

How should the dry eye syndrome be treated?

With iatrogenic problems, a change of drug may be all that is required. When the dry eye is associated with the ageing process, the condition is often intractable and palliative treatment with artificial tears is necessary.

Which tear substitute is best?

There has been little comparative data on the available tear substitutes but surprisingly in a recent double-blind cross-over study a hypotonic (150 m Osm/l) solution was preferred to solutions of higher tonicity. Hypromellose, macrogol, polivinyl alcohol and dextran are commonly used viscosifying agents but there is little data to base comparisons of performance on. The preservative system is also variable and benzalkonium chloride, chlorhexidine and chlorobutanol and sorbic acid are current alternatives. Chlorhexidine is often regarded as less irritant than the quaternary ammonium compounds, in the cornea. Claims that sorbic acid is a less irritant eye-drop preservative are still inadequately validated by use experience.

Are eye ointments useful for dry eyes?

Eye ointments may be useful for night-time use. Their day-time use may be uncomfortable and may lead to destabilization of the tear film and impairment of visual acuity.

Is inclusion of acetylcysteine in tear substitutes useful?

Acetylcysteine is a mucolytic agent and should theoretically be useful when there is excessive mucus present. There is as yet insufficient data to validate its usefulness in the dry eye syndrome.

Precautions and when to refer

 If vision is impaired.

 Cases not relieved by tear substitutes.

Product options

Hypotears Eye Drops (macrogol 8000, polivinyl alcohol)

Isopto Alkaline (hypromellose)

Isopto Plain (hypromellose)

Minims Artificial Tears (hydroxyethycellulose)

Optrex Dry Eye Therapy Eye Drops (hypromellose)

Refresh Ophthalmic Solution (polivinyl alcohol)

Sno Tears Eye Drops (polivinyl alcohol)

Tears Naturale (dixtran 70, hypromellose)

Viscotears Eye Drops (carbomer 940)

Dry mouth

What causes dry mouth?

Impaired salivary secretion is usually the cause of dry mouth (Xerostomia). However, the mechanisms for the decreased salivary output are often complex and unclear. The fact that the elderly suffer more commonly from dry mouth than do younger individuals suggests that decreased salivary function may be part of the ageing process. Factors which affect salivary output include: (1) emotional stress, (2) centrally-acting drugs including anticholinergics, opiates and levodopa, (3) central nervous pathology, (4) local factors affecting salivary function including

Table 11   Drugs which may cause dry mouth.

Amiloride	Emopronium bromide	Nortriptyline
Amitriptyline	Etretinate	Orphenadrine
Atropine	Flavoxate	Oxypertine
Azatadine	Fluphenazine	Pargyline
Benzhexol	Fluspirilene	Pericyazine
Benztropine	Hydroxyzine	Phenazocine
Biperiden	Hyoscine butylbromide	Phenelzine
Bromocriptine	Imipramine	Phenindamine
Busulphan	Indoramin	Phenylbutazone
Carbamazepine	Ipratropium	Pirenzepine
Chlormezanone	Iproniazid	Poldine
Chlorpromazine	Isocarboxazid	Potassium clorazepate
Clemastine	Isotretinoin	Prazosin
Clobazam	Ketamine	Prochlorporazine
Clomipramine	Ketotifen	Procyclidine
Clonazepam	Levodopa	Promazine
Clonidine	Lofepramine	Propantheline
Cyclizine	Maprotiline	Pyridostigmine
Cyproheptadine	Mazindol	Sulphasalazine
Desipramine	Mepyramine	Suxamethonium
Dexamphetamine	Methixene	Thioridazine
Dicyclomine	Methotrimeprazine	Tranycypromine
Diethylpropion	Methyldopa	Trazodone
Diphenylpyraline	Nabilone	Triamterene
Disopyramide	Nadolol	Trifluoperazine
Dothiepin	Nalbuphine	Trimeprazine
Doxapram	Nefopam	Trimipramine
Doxepin	Neostigmine	Viloxazine
Edrephonium	Nomifensine	

Sjögren's syndrome, infection and irradiation and (5) fluid imbalance induced by dehydration, organic pathology or drugs. Table 11 lists drugs which may cause dry mouth, based on literature or theoretical considerations.

What are the potential complications of xerostomia?

Dysphagia or difficulty in swallowing is one of the most distressing complications of dry mouth. Halitosis also develops and provides evidence for increased microbial concentration. Persistence of the problem leads to oral infections including dental caries, periodontitis and fungal infections.

What products are available for the treatment of dry mouth?

Artificial saliva, which may contain polymers (e.g. methylcellulose), polyhydric compounds (e.g. glycerol, sorbitol), fruit acids (e.g. citric acid) and electrolytes, is often recommended.

Precautions and when to refer

(R) Patients with persistent thirst (diabetes mellitus).

(R) Patients receiving one of the drugs which may cause dry mouth.

(!) Recommend scrupulous dental hygiene in these patients.

(!) Do not recommend sucking sweets as a cure.

Product options

Glandosane Spray (carmellose sodium, sorbitol, electrolytes)
Luborant Spray (carmellose sodium, sorbitol, electroytes)
Saliva Orthana Spray (gastric mucin, xylitol, sodium fluoride)
Saliva Orthana Lozenges (mucin, xylitol, sorbitol)
Salivace Spray (carmellose sodium, xylitol, electrolytes)
Saliveze Spray (carmellose sodium, electrolytes)
Salivix Pastilles (malic acid)

Dysmenorrhoea

What is dysmenorrhoea?

Dysmenorrhoea or period pain is caused by excessive production of prostaglandins by the uterus during menstruation. These prostaglandins sensitize pain receptors to other pain-inducing substances present in the menstrual fluid. Associated symptoms may include nausea, headache, fatigue, weakness and dizziness.

Precautions and when to refer_____

(R) Incapacitating; poor relief with ibuprofen

(R) Worsening from month to month.

(R) Presence of fever.

(R) Abnormal discharge or bleeding.

(R) Patient on IUD.

(R) Abdominal pain unrelated to period.

(!) See under analgesics.

(!) General recommendations

Ibuprofen is the agent of first choice in dysmenorrhoea unless the patient

(1) is hypersensitive to aspirin or NSAIDS;
(2) has a history of gastro-intestinal irritation, notably bleeding or ulceration;
(3) suffers from renal problems;
(4) is receiving a drug which may interact with it.

Under such circumstances paracetamol is usually acceptable.
   Antispasmodics such as hyoscine-N-butylbromide (Buscopan) and hyoscine

hydrobromide (present in Feminax) add little to the effect of the minor analgesics in dysmenorrhoea.

Herbal products for dysmenorrhoea are essentially placebos.

Selected product options

Any single-agent ibuprofen-containing analgesic
Paracetamol-containing products

Ear problems

What causes ear-wax and does it serve any purpose?

Ear-wax (cerumen) consists of secretions from the numerous sebaceous and apocrine glands lining the external auditory canal. Other entrapped debris includes exfoliated surface cells and hairs. The cerumen is continuously secreted to provide a protective barrier against infection. In addition to waxes, the acidic secretions include immunoglobulins and lysosymes. Under normal circumstances, desiccated cerumen is moved outwards by jaw movements during speech and masticatory action, to be removed during normal cleansing of the outer ear. In some individuals excessively cohesive cerumen is produced and accumulation takes place. This may be stimulated by mechanical interference of the minor portion of the ear canal and infection. Plugging then results and normal hearing is reversibly impaired.

How can excess ear-wax be removed?

Excess ear-wax may be removed by careful mechanical action. However, because this may further complicate the problem, alternative methods are more appropriate. Mild cases resolve spontaneously by discouraging mechanical probing of the inner canal. More severe cases benefit from ear-drops which soften and emulsify or dissolve the excess wax for subsequent drainage (see below). The most recalcitrant cases will need syringing.

Rectified *camphor oil* which is made up of the lighter fractions of the oil obtained as a by-product of camphor extraction helps to soften cerumen and may in addition have some counter-irritant properties. *Fixed oils* such as arachis oil (peanut oil) and almond oil are common basic materials for cerumen-softening drops. Cerumen includes hydrophobic components so that partial dissolution and softening by the oils can be expected although there is some evidence to show that water-soluble bases may be advantageous (see below under sodium dioctyl sulphosuccinate). Ethylene oxide-polyoxypropylene glycol condensate possesses surface active properties and may therefore help the ear drop base and/or active ingredient to penetrate the waxy matrix more rapidly. The advantages and disadvantages of its inclusion are similar to those discussed under sodium dioctyl sulphosuccinate.

Glycerol or glycerin, in addition to being used as the base for ear drops, is also widely recommended on its own for softening cerumen and some clinicians in fact claim that it may be as effective as any other preparation for this purpose. The inclusion of paradichlorobenzene, a compound which seems to be a better insecticide than a ceruminolytic agent, in some ear drops is irrational. The toxicity of the compound is such that a maximum permissible atmospheric concentration (75 ppm) is imposed. Serious allergic reactions have also been reported following contact with paradichlorobenzene.

Penetration of the ear drop instilled into the cerumen matrix is a prerequisite to cerumen softening and its eventual removal. The use of a surfactant such as sodium dioctyl sulphosuccinate (SDSS) is therefore a logical step although there is still doubt as to whether it is useful. Thus, in one study it was found that an ear drop containing 5% SDSS was no more effective than the maize oil base on its own. A subsequent study, however, indicated that when 5% SDSS, formulated in a water-miscible base, was used (Waxsol), the product was better than Cerumol. The end-point used to assess the product was the volume of water required to remove impacted wax by syringing.

These two studies taken together would therefore indicate that SDSS should be formulated in a water-miscible base. This is supported by the observation that *in vitro* Waxsol produced a more rapid disintegration of extracted cerumen than did Dioctyl ear drops which were formulated in an oily base. Some clinicians, however, feel that an oil base is preferable, although the manufacturers appear to have been sufficiently convinced to reformulate Dioctyl drops in a water-miscible base.

What is otitis externa?

Otitis externa is caused by infection of the outer ear. While otitis externa is not usually a serious complaint, it can incapacitate, and professional swimmers and divers are particularly at risk. Prevention is therefore important. The use of pro-tective gear to avoid the introduction of water into the ear is a useful protective measure. Dehydrating solvents such as ethyl alcohol and the glycols have also been recommended. Spirit Ear Drops BPC may be suitable for this purpose. Acetic acid ear drops are also thought useful both to reverse the disruption of the acid mantle of the external auditory canal and to provide antimicrobial cover. The use of boric acid drops is more debatable and should preferably not be recommended. Aluminium acetate drops which exert an astringent action may be useful in controlling the inflammation.

Antibacterial treatment of otitis externa, in the presence of perforation of the tympanic membrane, may increase the risk of drug-induced deafness if topical agents such as chlorhexidine and aminoglycosides are used. Occasionally, otitis externa becomes persistent, particularly in diabetics. Therefore, diabetes should be excluded in patients presenting with chronic otitis externa or recurrent boils in the ear.

What is otitis media?

Acute otitis media or inflammation of the middle ear is particularly common in children and often accompanies upper respiratory tract infections. Otalgia and fever are common symptoms of the disease although chronic otitis media may be totally asymptomatic. The Eustachian tube maintains atmospheric pressure within the middle ear. Viral or microbial attack leads to inflammation of the tube. The pressure equilibration mechanism is disrupted and negative pressures build up in the middle ear. The force generated produces transudation of fluid into the cavity and a good growth medium is therefore provided by the effusion, although its immunoglobulin content no doubt exerts a protective action.

There is still controversy about the microbiology of middle ear effusions in otitis media. *Streptococcus pneumonia* and *Haemophilus influenza* have consistently been frequent isolates in early studies. A recent study, however, indicated that although this was so there was no significant difference between the frequency with which these micro-organisms were isolated from otitis media effusions and from a control group. Viruses and *Streptococcus pyogenes* were, however, much more commonly isolated in the presence of otitis media. An even more recent study showed that viruses were more often implicated in otitis media with effusion than were bacteria. The more severe infections are sometimes thought to be of bacterial origin but over a quarter of infections are preceded or accompanied by upper respiratory viral infections.

If the condition is not causing undue stress within 48 hours, analgesics may be adequate. Oral analgesics are generally preferred although it has been claimed that topical analgesic ear drops may give faster relief. Self-treatment of otitis media is not justified as antibiotic cover may be required.

What do non-prescription analgesic and antibacterial ear drops contain and are they useful?

Chlorbutol (chlorbutanol) is a counter-irritant with antibacterial and anti-fungal properties and concentrations of up to 5% are used in ear drops. Choline salicylate has been claimed to have a more rapid onset of action when applied topically than oral aspirin or paracetamol in relieving ear-ache (otalgia). Phenazone or antipyrine is an analgesic compound which is now only very rarely used orally because of the recognition that the available alternatives, notably aspirin and paracetamol, are clearly superior both in terms of efficacy and safety. Topically, phenazone has no clear advantage over the salicylates and appears to be much more likely to induce skin sensitization.

Turpentine oil (oleum terebinthinae), an oil obtained by the distillation and rectification of the oleo-resin (turpentine) obtained from various species of pine trees (*Pinus pinaceae*), is included in some of the more popular ear drops, mainly for its counter-irritant properties. Turpentine oil has, however, been shown to be a relatively strong skin sensitizer. Propylene glycol-containing ear drops should be avoided but unfortunately, there is often no easy way of ascertaining the absence of this excipient in ear drops.

Hydrogen peroxide ear drops were at one time widely recommended for the softening of ear wax. Sodium bicarbonate drops, olive oil and almond oil are now thought to be better alternatives because of their relative inertness. The anti-bacterial but potentially irritant Phenol ear drops, especially in the presence of water, are also now less favoured than previously, for the same reason.

Are decongestants and antihistamines useful in otitis media?

Decongestants both alone and in combination with antihistamines are often recommended for the alleviation of symptoms associated with acute otitis media although there is still little evidence for their effectiveness. In one study a pseudoephedrine and carbinoxamine maleate combination was found to produce more rapid equalization of middle ear pressures than a placebo. In a second study chlorpheniramine maleate was found to be useful, but subsequent studies have not always confirmed the usefulness of either the decongestants or the antihistamines.

Precautions and when to refer

(R) Refer all cases of earache, especially with children.

(R) If patients complain of dizziness or liquid discharges.

(!) Avoid analgesic and anaesthetic ear drops as they may mask infections.

(!) Avoid phenazone, turpentine oil and chlorbutol as they are more likely to sensitize.

(!) Benzocaine has not been proven to be either safe or effective on topical application.

(!) Check for possible ototoxic drugs, notably gentamicin, streptomycin, kanamycin, ethacrynic acid, frusemide, salicylates, quinine and chloroquine and refer as appropriate.

Product options

Exterol Ear Drops (urea-hydrogen peroxide complex, glycerin)
Molcer Ear Drops (docusate sodium)

Otex Ear Drops (urea hydrogen peroxide)
Waxsol Ear Drops (docusate sodium)

Second-line products
Audax Ear Drops (chlorine, salicylate, glycerin)
Cerumol Ear Drops (chlorbutol, arachis oil, dichlorobenzene)
Earex (camphor, almond oil, arachis oil)
Wax Wane Ear Drops (turpentine oil 15%)

Eczema

What is eczema?

The term eczema is used to describe a variety of inflammatory skin conditions with diverse causes and presentations. The condition may be acute, subacute or chronic. Itch is almost invariably present. Other common features include crusting, erythema, exudation, lichenification (thickening with striae) and scaling.

Causative factors include occlusive contact with urine or faeces (napkin dermatitis), stasis (gravitational eczema) and contact with allergenic substances (e.g. nickel contact dermatitis). Often no causative factor can be established and the term atopic eczema is used. The term dermatitis is used synonymously with eczema.

How should eczema be managed?

Clearly when a causative factor can be identified its removal is the most appropriate treatment. Dry, fissured and scaly lesions are best treated with emollients. Allergic contact and irritant dermatitis can be treated with hydrocortisone cream or ointment during the acute phases and subsequently with emollients. Napkin dermatitis is not a licensed indication for non-prescription hydrocortisone creams or ointments. When thickening of the skin is evident, a salicylic acid or coal tar based product may be helpful. Use of emulsifying ointment as a substitute may bring about a significant improvement. There is some limited clinical data to suggest that oral gammolenic acid (evening primrose oil) may be useful in eczema. Topical gammolenic acid products are probably no more useful than cheaper emollients.

Why is hydrocortisone useful in irritant or contact dermatitis?

Irritant or contact and atopic dermatitis responds well to topical hydrocortisone. Hydrocortisone has an antimitotic activity. This and its anti-inflammatory and anti-pruritic actions contribute to the drug's effectiveness in this condition.

What are the potential adverse effects of hydrocortisone?

Excessive systemic concentrations of hydrocortisone lead to severe adverse reactions and Cushing's syndrome, with the development of a bull-like torso, is a classical presentation with chronic overdosing. Excessive hydrocortisone levels also interfere with lymphoid tissue and therefore integrity of the immune system is impaired. When applied topically, suppression of the immune system leads to an increased likelihood of infection. Telangiectasia has been observed following application to eye-lids but skin toxicity, in general, is much less pronounced with hydrocortisone than with the more potent steroids. Applications to the eyes or face, the anogenital region or to broken or infected skin including acne, cold sores and athlete's foot, are contraindicated for non-prescription use. Use of the hydrocortisone products in children under 10 years and in pregnancy is also cautioned against. Table 12 lists OTC indications for topical hydrocortisone products.

Table 12   Licensed indications for topical hydrocortisone products*.

Acne	Itching
Allergic dermatitis	Lupus erythematosis
Contact dermatitis	Nappy rash
Dermatitis	Neurodermatitis
Eczema	Otitis externa
Erythema	Pompholyx
Exfoliative dermatitis	Prickly heat
Haemorrhoids	Pruritus
Hyperkeratetic lesions	Psoriasis
Inflammatory skin conditions	Rashes
Insect bites	Seborrhoeic dermatitis
Intertrigo	Sunburn
Irritant dermatitis	

*Non-prescription indications in italics.

How does hydrocortisone work?

Hydrocortisone (cortisol) is the main glucocorticosteroid secreted by the adrenal cortex, accounting for over 95% of the glucocorticosteroid activity of the adrenal cortex and participating in carbohydrate, protein and fat metabolism. Topical hydrocortisone is mainly used for its anti-pruritic and anti-inflammatory activity. Until recently inhibition of phospholipase A_2 leading to reduced availability of free arachidonic acid and hence inhibition of prostaglandin synthesis was the most widely held view about the mechanism of the anti-inflammatory and anti-pruritic action of the corticosteroids.

More recent evidence suggests that this view is no longer tenable. It is now thought that the corticosteroids bind to steroid receptors to form a steroid-receptor complex. This then undergoes allosteric changes to become activated thereby acquiring affinity for nuclear structures. Within the nucleus, the complex initiates transcription of specific mRNA which then translocates to the ribosomes to direct the synthesis of regulatory peptides. These mediate the cellular responses observed. Among the many activities of those peptides are a reduction in lymphokine synthesis, a modulatory effect on the synthesis of enzymes involved in prostaglandin synthesis and the induction of the synthesis of inhibitory proteins such as lipocortin and interleukin-1.

Is *Staphylococcus aureus* colonisation important in eczema?

Staphylococcus aureus

Several authors have drawn attention to the fact that *Staphylococcus aureus* is found more frequently and in larger numbers in the skin of eczema patients when compared to normal subjects. Some surveys suggest that more than 90% of eczema patients with chronic lichenified plaques carried the pathogen and that in the acute, exudative form of the disease, the organism can essentially always be recovered at densities exceeding 18.7 million per cm^2. In the normal population, normal skin carriage rate is of the order of 10%. It has been suggested that *Staphylococcus aureus* may have an unusual ability to adhere to atopic corneocytes and that a particular protein (Protein A) may be responsible for this. Indeed there are now good experimental data to indicate that *S. aureus* adheres specifically to atopic cells. An early theory that sebaceous or eccrine secretions were different in eczema patients when compared to those in normal patients has now largely been abandoned.

Is the association between *Staphylococcus aureus* and eczema of pathological significance?

The most prevalent view appears to be that *Staphylococcus aureus* does not initiate eczema but it may prolong episodes of eczema by promoting inflammation.

Current theory suggests that when *S. aureus* colonise eczematous skin, they produce exotoxins which trigger cells of the immune system to activate and perpetuate inflammation. Indeed, repeated occlusive exposures of skin to cell wall protein A of *S. aureus* leads to an inflammatory response.

With inflammation, there is a leakage of white cells into the deeper skin (dermis) and fluid accumulation (spongiosis). As inflammation worsens, vesicle formation follows. The vesicles are disrupted with scratching and weeping and exudation follow. Eventually the exudates dry up leading to crust formation. As the cycle repeats itself, the skin becomes thickened (lichenification) and the areas affected (e.g. hands) may lose flexibility. Any moist area will, of course, provide further opportunities for microbial overgrowth.

Does it help to institute antimicrobial chemotherapy?

Antimocrobial chemotherapy is used for the management of acute exacerbations of the disease. Some data on topical mupiromycin suggests that by reducing bacterial count, clinical severity of eczema can be reduced. Complete elimination of dermal *S. aureus* is not possible.

There has yet not been any systematic evaluation of the efficacy of antiseptic formulations against *S. aureus* in atopic eczema and coupling of the results to clinical changes. Some have suggested that Candida albicans (a yeast commonly associated with thrush) and pityrosponum species (associated with dandruff) may also be implicated in atopic eczema, but current consensus is that they are unimportant in the disease.

Precautions and when to refer

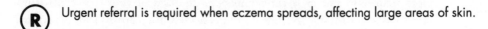 Urgent referral is required when eczema spreads, affecting large areas of skin.

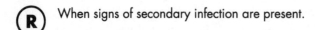 When signs of secondary infection are present.

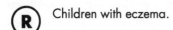 Children with eczema.

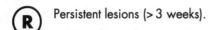 Persistent lesions (> 3 weeks).

Products options

Alcoderm Cream (liquid paraffin)

Alpha Keri Bath (liquid paraffin, soluble wool fat)

Aquadrate Cream (Urea)

Aveeno Bath Oil (colloidal oatmeal)

Aveeno Cream (colloidal oatmeal)

Balneum Liquid Bath (soya oil)

Balneum Plus Liquid Bath (soya oil, lauromacrogols)

Bath E45 Oil (cetyl dimethicone)

Calmund Cream (urea, lactic acid)

Cream E45 (liquid paraffin, white soft paraffin, lanolin)

Dermamist Spray (white soft paraffin, liquid paraffin, fractionated coconut oil – FLAMMABLE)

Diprobath Bath Additive (isopropyl myristate, liquid paraffin)

Diprobase Cream (liquid paraffin, white soft paraffin, cetomacrogol, cetostearylalcohol)

Emmolate Bath Oil (acetylated wood alcohols, liquid paraffin)

Emulsiderm Liquid Emulsion (liquid paraffin, isopropyl myristate)

Hydromol Cream (liquid paraffin, sodium pyrollidone carboxylate)

Hydromol Emollient (isopropyl myristate)

Infaderm Oil (liquid paraffin, almond oil)

Imuderm Oil (liquid paraffin, almond oil)

Kamillosan Ointment (chamomile extract)

Keri Lotion (liquid paraffin, lanolin oil)

Lacticase Lotion (lactic acid, sodium pyrollidone carboxylate)

Neutrogena Dermatological Cream (glycerol)

Nutraplus Cream (urea)

Oilatum Bath Additive (liquid paraffin)

Oilatum Gel (liquid paraffin)

Oilatum Plus (triclosan, benzalkonium chloride, liquid paraffin)

Oilatum Shower Emollient Gel (liquid paraffin)

Oilatum Skin Therapy Bath Additive (liquid paraffin)

Ultrabase Cream (liquid paraffin, white soft paraffin)

Unguentum Merck (hydro-lipophilic base)

Vaseline Dermacase Cream (dimethicone, white soft paraffin)

Evening primrose oil

Is evening primrose oil useful in eczema?

Evening primrose oil (EPO) is in fact licensed for the symptomatic relief of eczema, thus suggesting that there is indeed some information supporting its use for that purpose. In one of the first studies investigating the usefulness of EPO in eczema, both patients and doctors reported an improvement in the symptoms of eczema after 3 weeks' treatment with 500 mg EPO capsules. In a subsequent study, eczematous itch was relieved by low dose EPO, while scaling required 2–3 g of oil daily for improvement to be detectable. However, other studies have been less promising and there is a need to better define the oil's effectiveness in eczema. Oral therapy appears to be better than topical EPO therapy which appears to be no better than placebo.

Is evening primrose oil effective in premenstrual syndrome?

Premenstrual syndrome (PMS) or premenstrual tension (PMT) is an extremely complex condition, probably of multifactorial origin. However, some authors are of the opinion that abnormalities in prostaglandin synthesis are involved, probably through changes in prolactin levels. A recent meta-analysis suggests that EPO is no better than placebo in PMS.

Is evening primrose oil effective in lowering blood cholesterol?

Gamma-linolenic acid is effective in lowering blood cholesterol. Since the enzyme which converts linoleic acid to gamma-linolenic acid appears to be deficient in hypercholesterolaemia, EPO supplements should theoretically be useful but are expensive and efficacy has not been demonstrated. Alternative methods of reducing blood cholesterol, notably alterations in the diet, are likely to be much more rewarding.

Is evening primrose oil effective in multiple sclerosis?

Multiple sclerosis is a poorly understood disease affecting the brain and spinal cord. The myelin sheath around nerve fibres is destroyed and prognosis is poor. Linoleic acid appears to retard the progression of the disease. Linolenic acid and hence EPO have also been suggested but their value has not been adequately tested.

Precautions and when to refer

 Care with patients with a history of epilepsy.

Branded products containing evening primrose oil or starflower oil

Evening Primrose Oil
Efamol Original Capsules
Efamol Original High Strength Capsules
Efamol Original Liquid
EPOC 1000 Capsules

Sanatogen Evening Primrose Oil Capsules
Seven Seas Chewable Evening Primrose
  Oil Capsules

Evening Primrose Oil + Fish Oil
Efamol Marine Capsules

Efamol Marine High Strength Capsules

Evening Primrose Oil + Multivitamins
Efamol Plus Capsules

Sanatogen Multivitamins Plus Evening
  Primrose Oil

Starflower Oil
Sanatogen Starflower Oil Capsules
Seven Seas Evening Primrose Oil Plus
  Starflower Oil

Starflower Oil Capsules

Fish oils and garlic oil

What is the rationale for the use of fish oils for preventing cardiovascular disease?

Biochemically, fish oils have attracted much attention because of their eicosapentaenoic acid and docosahexaenoic acid contents, while evening primrose oil has

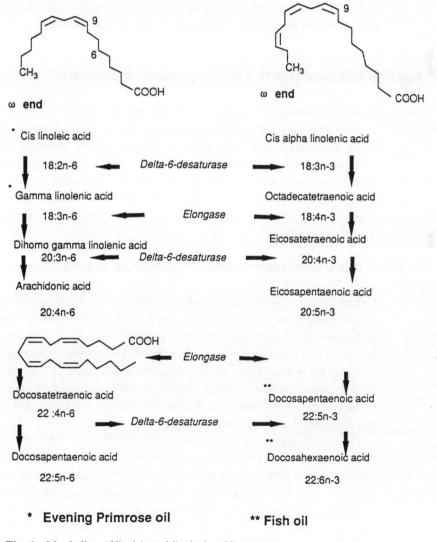

* Cis linoleic acid

18:2n-6 ← Delta-6-desaturase → Cis alpha linolenic acid 18:3n-3

* Gamma linolenic acid

18:3n-6 ← Elongase → Octadecatetraenoic acid 18:4n-3

Dihomo gamma linolenic acid
20:3n-6 ← Delta-6-desaturase → Eicosatetraenoic acid 20:4n-3

Arachidonic acid
20:4n-6

Eicosapentaenoic acid
20:5n-3

← Elongase → Docosapentaenoic acid 22:5n-3

Docosatetraenoic acid
22:4n-6 → Delta-6-desaturase →

Docosahexaenoic acid
22:6n-3

Docosapentaenoic acid
22:5n-6

* **Evening Primrose oil**   ** **Fish oil**

Fig. 6 Metabolism of linoleic and linolenic acids.

stimulated research because of its unusually high gamma-linolenic acid content. Their inter-relationships are shown in Figure 6.

Epidemiological data clearly show that there is a relationship between cardiovascular disease and saturated fat intake. Communities with higher fish consumption rates also have lower death rates from coronary disease, while consumption of fish oil has been shown to cause a reduction in thromboxane A(production, a potent platelet aggregator, and an increase in PGI_3, a potent inhibitor of platelet aggregation. Fish oil also causes a lowering in blood viscosity, plasma triglycerides, very low density lipoprotein and plasma fibrinogen. All of those changes are thought to decrease the likelihood of developing cardiovascular disease. The data are sufficiently convincing for a number of drug regulatory authorities to license the use of fish-oils for a number of indications. In the UK, fish oils are approved for the reduction of plasma triglycerides in severe hypertriglyceridaemia and in those at special risk of ischaemic disease and/or pancreatitis.

Are fish oils useful in the management of psoriasis?

Psoriatic plaques show increased levels of arachidonic acid, 12 hydroxyeicosatetraenoic acid and leukotriene B_4. Potent cyclo-oxygenase inhibitors which shunt arachidonic acid towards the lipoxygenase pathways may make psoriasis worse. It is postulated that fish oils, with their eicosapentaenoic and docosahexaenoic acids contents, restore the normal balance and correct the underlying abnormality. Some small trials have shown some beneficial effects including less itching, erythema and scaling, but confirmation is still required.

Are fish oils useful for treating rheumatoid arthritis?

Fish oil supplementation inhibits cyclo-oxygenase conversion of arachidonic acid to inflammatory series 2 prostanoids and to leukotriene B_4, a potent chemotaxin. Instead the less inflammatory series 3 prostanoids and series 5 leukotrienes are formed. There is some evidence to show that fish oils improve morning stiffness, grip strength and number of tender joints, when given orally to patients suffering from rheumatoid arthritis. Such improvements are accompanied by improvements in the biochemical markers of the disease. For example, erythrocyte sedimentation rate is improved and leukotriene B_4 levels fall.

The clinical improvements achieved so far with fish oils are, however, relatively modest when compared with traditional non-steroidal anti-inflammatory drugs and the toxicological profiles of the oils following long-term administration have yet to be defined. The reported beneficial effects of the fish oils suggest that a change in diet from one rich in red meats to one containing more fish is justified. The results also support some cautious use of fish oil products by rheumatoid arthritic patients. They do not as yet justify consumption of large doses of the oils.

What is garlic oil promoted for?

Garlic has been promoted for a wide range of illnesses ranging from cancer to heart disease and as a general tonic. Perhaps its most widespread use is as prophylactic against cardiovascular disease because of its claimed antilipidaemic, antioxidant, antiplatelet and fibrinolytic activities. However, much of the proposed rationale for its use is based on the association between low rate of cardiovascular disease and diets rich in garlic (mediterranean diets).

Is garlic effective as a cardioprotective agent?

Recent meta-analyses suggest that garlic may reduce choloesterol levels and blood-pressure but publication bias appears to be a problem. To date there have not been any trials of sufficient power to evaluate whether garlic guards against cardiovascular disease or its clinical consequences. Reducing fat intake and smoking and increasing physical activity are still the best advice for those trying to avoid cardiovascular disease. The jury is still out on the value of garlic.

Branded products containing garlic oil

Höfels Cod Liver Oil and Garlic Perles Capsules
Höfels Cardiomax Garlic Capsules
Höfels Odourless Neo Garlic Perles Capsules
Höfels Vitamin C and Garlic Capsules
Sanatogen Once a Day Garlic Perles Capsules
Sanatogen Cod Liver Oil with Garlic Capsules
Seven Seas Odourless Garlic Perles
Seven Seas Cod Liver Oil and Odourless Garlic Capsules

Branded products containing fish oils

Efamol Plus Fish Oils and Co-enzyme Q Capsules
Sanatogen Pure Fish Oils Capsules
Seven Seas Pulse High Strength Pure Fish Oils
Seven Seas Pulse High Strength Pure Fish Oils Capsules

Food allergy

What is food allergy?

In common usage food allergy refers to any hypersensitivity or abnormal reaction to specific food items. Biochemically, however, food allergy is distinct from the other two food hypersensitivity reactions, food intolerance and food aversion. Food allergy is immunologically-based and is associated with a raised blood level of IgE and with the presence of IgE antibodies to food components. It has been suggested that in the presence of food allergy, an IgE-mediated mechanism alters the permeability of the gastric mucosa to allow entry of the antigens and the formation of immune complexes.

Food aversion is usually psychosomatic in nature. Anorexia nervosa is a well-publicized variant of the problem. The subject develops symptoms of revulsion at the sight and smell of food and therefore eventually suffers from malnutrition and wasting of tissues. Food intolerance is characterized by classical symptoms of food hypersensitivity but although the symptoms can be reproducibly elicited by exposure to the offending foods, no immunological or psychological bases can be uncovered. The underlying mechanism may be a deficiency of an enzyme such as lactase in lactose intolerance, a non-specific histamine-releasing effect as is seen in strawberry hypersensitivity or an abnormal response to a normally well-tolerated substance as in spice intolerance.

How common is food hypersensitivity?

Very wide estimates of prevalence of food hypersensitivity are reported in the literature. One study suggested that between 0.3% to 20% of children suffer or have suffered from symptoms of food intolerance. In a more recent study, 3% of the children surveyed were perceived as being food hypersensitive.

What is the best way to avoid food allergy?

Surprisingly recent data suggests that dietary manipulations are probably not the most effective way of avoiding food allergies. Instead avoidance of early contact with known allergens appears to be more rewarding in this respect. Avoidance of birth during the heavy pollen season and the dust-mite season, avoidance of pets and delay in introducing mixed solids are thought to be prophylactic against food allergies.

Is avoidance of food allergens by the mother helpful in preventing food intolerance in the newborn?

In utero sensitization to milk is known to occur with unknown frequency and some authorities recommend avoidance of the major food allergens during the last 2 months of pregnancy. The value of this approach is unknown.

What causes food aversion during pregnancy?

Little is known about this but one study suggested that mothers who subsequently gave birth to children showing intolerance to cow's milk tended to suffer more commonly from food aversion and nausea during pregnancy.

Is 3-month colic in babies a sign of milk hypersensitivity?

Colic in babies often appears to be food-related because of the predominance of abdominal symptoms. However, it is not clear how many cases, if any, can be ascribed to milk hypersensitivity (see also section on indigestion).

Is food hypersensitivity genetically determined?

Allergic reactions are certainly more common in children of atopic parents and a link between gluten sensitivity and HLAB8/W3 has been suggested. However in general, the mode of inheritance of food sensitivity, if present, is unclear.

What are the typical symptoms of food hypersensitivity?

Several syndromes may be observed. In some cases there is immediate inflammation and general irritation of the buccal mucosa accompanied or followed by nausea, vomiting and/or abdominal pain. Diarrhoea and excessive abdominal bloating may also be obvious. In other cases, gastro-intestinal symptoms are not apparent but instead symptoms resembling those of hay-fever emerge. Other symptoms of allergy such as asthma, eczema and joint pains may also be seen. Migraine, which is often attributed to the tyramine content of the offending foods, may also develop.

What do the E numbers of food additives refer to?

Food additives approved for use in the European Community are given a code number which is usually referred to as the E number. Thus, tartrazine has code number E102 and butylated hydroxytoluene has code number E321. The code numbers are now required, by the EEC regulations on food labelling, to be included on the packaging of the foods concerned. Table 13 lists the E number of additives commonly included in food formulations.

How important are food additives in initiating food hypersensitivity?

Food dyes, preservatives and other additives are commonly perceived as being responsible for food hypersensitivity reactions, an observation which some manufacturers have been quick to capitalize on. At one time, most orthodox scientists would have been sceptical of food additive-induced adverse reactions. This has gradually changed over the years so that now, most authorities would concede that hypersensitivity to at least some food additives is a real clinical entity. Tartrazine hypersensitivity is now a well-recognized problem although there is still much debate about the underlying mechanism. Hypersensitivity to benzoates, sulphur dioxide and antioxidants such as butylated hydroxyanisole and butylated hydroxytoluene are also being increasingly acknowledged.

Is hyperactivity a symptom of food hypersensitivity?

This is certainly an interesting hypothesis put forward by various authorities who recommend restricted diets in the management of food hypersensitivities. Although it is generally recognized that food hypersensitivity may manifest itself with a range of symptoms, some of which may be behavioural in nature, many are of the view that in only rare cases can hyperactivity be directly attributable to food hypersensitivity. Nonetheless specialist additive-free and salicylate-free diets are often promoted by various interested parties. The anagram SHIC (spoilt, hyperactive, intolerable children) may sometimes appear appropriate for describing the patients. Feingold suggests an incidence of up to 25% in some schools while others have estimated incidences, in the USA, of 3–10%, which are well above figures reported for the UK.

What is the Feingold diet?

The Feingold diet is an exclusion diet which eliminates salicylates and food-additives. Its rise to prominence is in the treatment of hyperactivity thought to be due to food hypersensitivity. Thus foods such as cucumber, oranges, apples and berries which contain naturally-occurring salicylate are excluded as are foods containing artificial additives. Despite trials showing the hyperactivity in children is not controlled by such diets, these remain popular.

If food-additives do not produce hyperactivity, do they cause any other adverse reactions?

There is now general agreement that some additives are certainly responsible for some adverse reactions. **Tartrazine** (E102) is perhaps the most thoroughly investigated example of a food additive which may produce symptoms mimicking allergic reactions. Other additives which have caused serious concern include cochineal (E120), erythrosine (E127), patent blue V (E131), indigo carmine (E132), copper complexes of chlorophyll and chlorophyllins (E141), greens (E142), caramel (E150) and annatto, bixin and norbixin (E160b). Some regulatory authorities now insist on the declaration of these particular dyes on product labels.

Is milk hypersensitivity a true allergy?

The evidence shows that in at least some of the patients hypersensitive to milk, the

underlying mechanism is immunological. In other cases such as in lactase deficiency, the condition is one of intolerance to components of milk rather than milk
allergy. A recent study suggested that there may be different sub-types of milk
allergy. In one group an immediate reaction (< 45 minutes after challenge), characterized by urticaria, is accompanied by an elevation of IgE milk-specific antibody
levels. In a second group, with an intermediate reaction (1–20 hours after challenge), vomiting and diarrhoea were the distressing symptoms with no elevation of
IgE-milk specific antibodies. In a third group with late reactions (> 20 hours) both
dermal and gastro-intestinal symptoms were obvious. Patients with the eczematous
symptoms still showed elevation in IgE-milk specific antibodies.

Can milk hypersensitivity be cured?

Most food hypersensitivity reactions, including milk hypersensitivity, resolve
spontaneously with time. The incidence of allergy is highest in the first few months of
life but gradually decreases with age. Close to half of all cases resolve within 3 years.

Is breast feeding a sure way of preventing milk-allergy?

An early study indicated that this was indeed the case. However, subsequent
studies have produced contradictory evidence. Indeed the presence of antigens in
breast milk has already been clearly demonstrated. Soy milk, which is often claimed
to be less allergenic, has also not lived up to manufacturers' claims. However,
although soy milk would not be preferable to standard cow's milk-based formulae
when breast-feeding is contraindicated, it is still a useful substitute in cases of
proven cow's milk allergy.

Can an infant develop allergies from its mother's milk?

There is indeed data to show that food antigens may be transferred to an infant
through its mother's milk. In one recent study an elimination diet improved eczema
in most of the 13 infants studied, while maternal challenge worsened the dermatitis
in 9/9 children with atopic dermatitis.

Is yoghurt safe for patients with milk allergy?

The micro-organisms (*Lactobacillus bulgaricus* and *Streptococcus thermophilus*) used
to prepare yoghurt produce lactases which hydrolyse lactose to absorbable glucose
and galactose. Symptoms of lactose intolerance are therefore inhibited. Yoghurt
should therefore be an acceptable milk-based food for individuals suffering from
lactase deficiency.

Why is food hypersensitivity more common in individuals who already suffer from other allergic diseases?

Food hypersensitivity reactions do indeed appear to be more common in atopic patients and recent work suggests that the reason may be due to allergen sensitization.

Precautions and when to refer

 Patients who are significantly underweight.

 Children showing abnormal physical or behavioural development.

Table 13   EEC serial numbers for food additives.

Numbers with the prefix 'E' are additives authorized on a permanent basis throughout the Community though not necessarily permitted by all Member States.

(Common alternative names for some additives are shown in bold type.)

E100	Curcumin
E101	Riboflavin (**lactoflavin**)
E101(a)	Riboflavin-5'-phosphate
E102	Tartrazine
E104	Quinoline Yellow
E107	Yellow 2G
E110	Sunset Yellow FCT (**orange Yellow S**)
E120	Cochineal (**carmine of cochineal or Carminic acid**)
E122	Carmoisine (**Azorubine**)
E123	Amaranth
E124	Ponceau 4R (**Cochineal Red A**)
E127	Erythrosine BS
E128	Red 2G
E131	Patent Blue V
E132	Indigo Carmine (**Indigotine**)
E133	Brilliant Blue FCF
E140	Chlorophyll
E141	Copper complexes of chlorophyll and chlorophyllins
E142	Green S (**Acid Brilliant Green BS or Lissamine Green**)
E150	Caramel
E151	Black PN (**Brilliant Black BN**)
E153	Carbon Black (**Vegetable Carbon**)
E154	Brown FK
E155	Brown HT (**Chocolate Brown HT**)
E160(a)	alpha-carotene, beta-carotene, gamma-carotene
E160(b)	annatto, bixin, norbixin
E160(c)	capsanthin (**Capsorubin**)
E160(d)	lycopene
E160(e)	beta-apo-8'-carotenal (C_{30})
E160(f)	ethyl ester of beta-apo-8'-carotenoic acid (C_{30})
E161(a)	Flavoxanthin
E161(b)	Lutein

Table 13   EEC serial numbers for food additives (*continued*).

E161(c)	Cryptoxanthin
E161(d)	Rubixanthin
E161(e)	Violaxanthin
E161(f)	Rhodoxanthin
E161(g)	Canthaxanthin
E162	Beetroot Red (**Betanin**)
E163	Anthocyanins
E170	Calcium carbonate
E171	Titanium dioxide
E172	Iron oxides, iron hydroxides
E173	Aluminium
E174	Silver
E175	Gold
E180	Pigment Rubine (**Lithol Rubine BK**)
E200	Sorbic acid
E201	Sodium sorbate
E202	Potassium sorbate
E203	Calcium sorbate
E210	Benzoic acid
E211	Sodium benzoate
E212	Potassium benzoate
E213	Calcium benzoate
E214	Ethyl 4–hydroxybenzoate (**Ethyl *para*-hydroxybenzoate**)
E215	Ethyl 4–hydroxybenzoate, sodium salt (**Sodium ethyl *para*-hydroxybenzoate**)
E216	Propyl 4–hydroxybenzoate (**Propyl *para*-hydroxybenzoate**)
E217	Propyl 4–hydroxybenzoate, sodium salt (**sodium propyl *para*-hydroxybenzoate**)
E218	Methyl 4–hydroxybenzoate (**Methyl *para*-hydroxybenzoate**)
E219	Methyl 4–hydroxybenzoate, sodium salt (**Sodium methyl *para*-hydroxybenzoate**)
E220	Sulphur dioxide
E221	Sodium sulphite
E222	Sodium hydrogen sulphite (**Sodium bisulphite**)
E223	Sodium metabisulphite
E224	Potassium metabisulphite
E226	Calcium sulphite
E227	Calcium hydrogen sulphite (**Calcium bisulphite**)
E230	Biphenyl (**Diphenyl**)
E231	2–Hydroxybiphenyl (**Orthophenylphenol**)
E232	Sodium biphenyl–2–yl oxide (**Sodium orthophenylphenate**)
E233	2–(Thiazol–4–yl) benzimadazole (**Thiabendazole**)
E234	Nisin
E239	Hexamine (**Hexamethylenetetramine**)
E249	Potassium nitrite
E250	Sodium nitrite
E251	Sodium nitrate
E252	Potassium nitrate
E260	Acetic acid
E261	Potassium acetate

Table 13   EEC serial numbers for food additives (*continued*).

E262	Sodium hydrogen diacetate
E262	Sodium acetate
E263	Calcium acetate
E270	Lactic acid
E280	Propionic acid
E281	Sodium propionate
E282	Calcium propionate
E283	Potassium propionate
E290	Carbon dioxide
E296	DL–Malic acid, L–Malic acid
E297	Fumaric acid
E300	L-Ascorbic acid
E301	Sodium L-ascorbate
E302	Calcium L-ascorbate
E304	6-*O*-Palmitoyl–L–ascorbic acid (**Ascorbyl palmitate**)
E306	Extracts of natural origin rich in tocopherols
E307	Synthetic *alpha*-tocopherol
E308	Synthetic *gamma*-tocopherol
E309	Synthetic *delta*-tocopherol
E310	Propyl gallate
E311	Octyl gallate
E312	Dodecyl gallate
E320	Butylated hydroxyanisol (**BHA**)
E321	Butylated hydroxytoluene (**BHT**)
E322	Lecithins
E325	Sodium lactate
E326	Potassium lactate
E327	Calcium lactate
E330	Citric acid
E331	Sodium dihydrogen citrate (*mono*Sodium citrate), *di*Sodium citrate, *tri*Sodium citrate
E332	Potassium dihydrogen citrate (*mono*Potassium citrate), *tri*Potassium citrate
E333	*mono*Calcium citrate, *di*Calcium citrate, *tri*Calcium citrate
E334	L-(+)-Tartaric acid
E335	*mono*Sodium L-(+)-tartrate, *di*Sodium L-(+)-tartrate
E336	*mono*Potassium L-(+)-tartrate (**Cream of tartar**), *di*Potassium L-(+)-tartrate
E337	Potassium sodium L-(+)-tartrate
E338	Orthophosphoric acid (**Phosphoric acid**)
E339	Sodium dihydrogen orthophosphate, *di*Sodium hydrogen orthophosphate, *tri*Sodium orthophosphate
E340	Potassium dihydrogen orthophosphate, *di*Potassium hydrogen orthophosphate, *tri*Potassium orthophosphate
E341	Calcium tetrahydrogen diorthophosphate, Calcium hydrogen orthophosphate, *tri*Calcium diorthophosphate
E350	Sodium malate, sodium hydrogen malate
E351	Potassium malate
E352	Calcium malate, calcium hydrogen malate
E353	Metatartaric acid

Table 13   EEC serial numbers for food additives (*continued*).

E355	Adipic acid
E363	Succinic acid
E370	I,4–Heptonolactone
E375	Nicotinic acid
E380	*tri*Ammonium citrate
E381	Ammonium ferric citrate
E385	Calcium disodium ethylenediamine- NNN'N' tetra-acetate **(Calcium disodium EDTA)**
E400	Alginic acid
E401	Sodium alginate
E402	Potassium alginate
E403	Ammonium alginate
E404	Calcium alginate
E405	Propane-1,2-diol alginate **(Propylene glycol alginate)**
E406	Agar
E407	Carrageenan
E410	Locust bean gum **(Carob gum)**
E412	Guar gum
E413	Tragacanth
E414	Gum arabic **(Acacia)**
E415	Xanthan gum
E416	Karaya gum
E420	Sorbitol, sorbitol syrup
E421	Mannitol
E422	Glycerol
E430	Polyoxyethylene (8) stearate
E431	Polyoxyethylene (40) stearate
E432	Polyoxyethylene (20) sorbitan monolaurate **(Polysorbate 20)**
E433	Polyoxyethylene (20) sorbitan mono-oleate **(Polysorbate 80)**
E434	Polyoxyethylene (20) sorbitan monopalmitate **(Polysorbate 40)**
E435	Polyoxyethylene (20) sorbitan monostearate **(Polysorbate 60)**
E436	Polyoxyethylene (20) sorbitan tristearate **(Polysorbate 65)**
E440(a)	Pectin
E440(b)	Amidated pectin
E442	Ammonium phosphatides
E450(a)	*di*Sodium dihydrogen diphosphate, *tri*Sodium diphosphate, *tetra*Sodium diphosphate, *tetra*Potassium diphosphate
E450(b)	*penta*Sodium triphosphate, *penta*Potassium triphosphate
E450(c)	Sodium polyphosphates, Potassium polyphosphates
E460	Microcrystalline cellulose, *Alpha*-cellulose **(Powdered cellulose)**
E461	Methylcellulose
E463	Hydroxypropylcellulose
E464	Hydroxypropylmethylcellulose
E465	Ethylmethylcellulose
E466	Carboxymethylcellulose, sodium salt **(CMC)**
E470	Sodium, potassium and calcium salts of fatty acids
E471	Mono- and di-glycerides of fatty acids
E472(a)	Acetic acid esters of mono- and di-glycerides of fatty acids
E472(b)	Lactic acid esters of mono- and di-glycerides of fatty acids **(Lactoglycerides)**

Table 13   EEC serial numbers for food additives (*continued*).

E472(c)	Citric acid esters of mono- and di-glycerides of fatty acids (**Citroglycerides**)
E472(e)	Mono- and diacetyltartaric acid esters of mono- and di-glycerides of fatty acids
E473	Sucrose esters of fatty acids
E474	Sucroglycerides
E475	Polyglycerol esters of fatty acids
E476	Polyglycerol esters of polycondensed fatty acids of castor oil (**Polyglycerol polyricinoleate**)
E477	Propane-1,2-diol esters of fatty acids
E478	Lactylated fatty acid esters of glycerol and propane-1,2-diol
E481	Sodium stearoyl-2-lactylate
E482	Calcium stearoyl-2-lactylate
E483	Stearyl tartrate
E491	Sorbitan monostearate
E492	Sorbitan tristearate
E493	Sorbitan monolaurate
E494	Sorbitan mono-oleate
E495	Sorbitan monopalmitate
E500	Sodium carbonate, Sodium hydrogen carbonate (**Bicarbonate of soda**), Sodium sesquicarbonate
E501	Potassium carbonate, Potassium hydrogen carbonate
E503	Ammonium carbonate, Ammonium hydrogen carbonate
E504	Magnesium carbonate
E507	Hydrochloric acid
E508	Potassium chloride
E509	Calcium chloride
E510	Ammonium chloride
E513	Sulphuric acid
E514	Sodium sulphate
E515	Potassium sulphate
E516	Calcium sulphate
E518	Magnesium sulphate
E524	Sodium hydroxide
E525	Potassium hydroxide
E526	Calcium hydroxide
E527	Ammonium hydroxide
E528	Magnesium hydroxide
E529	Calcium Oxide
E530	Magnesium oxide
E535	Sodium ferrocyanide (**Sodium hexacyanoferrate (II)**)
E536	Potassium ferrocyanide (**Potassium hexacyanoferrate (II)**)
E540	*di*Calcium diphosphate
E541	Sodium aluminium phosphate
E542	Edible bone phosphate
E544	Calcium polyphosphates
E545	Ammonium polyphosphates
E551	Silicon dioxide (**Silica**)
E552	Calcium silicate
E553(a)	Magnesium silicate synthetic, Magnesium trisilicate
E553(b)	Talc

Table 13 EEC serial numbers for food additives (*continued*).

E554	Aluminium sodium silicate
E556	Aluminium calcium silicate
E558	Bentonite
E559	Kaolin
E570	Stearic acid
E572	Magnesium stearate
E575	D-Glucono-1,5-lactone (**Glucono *delta*-lactone**)
E576	Sodium gluconate
E577	Potassium gluconate
E578	Calcium gluconate
E620	L-glutamic acid
E621	Sodium hydrogen L-glutamate (*mono***Sodium glutamate or MSG**)
E622	Potassium hydrogen L-glutamate (*mono***Potassium glutamate**)
E623	Calcium dihydrogen *di*-L-glutamate (**Calcium glutamate**)
E627	Guanosine 5'-(disodium phosphate) (**Sodium guanylate**)
E631	Inosine 5'-(disodium phosphate) (**Sodium inosinate**)
E635	Sodium 5'-ribonucleotide
E636	Maltol
E637	Ethyl maltol
E900	Dimethylpolysiloxane
E901	Beeswax
E903	Carnauba wax
E904	Shellac
E905	Mineral hydrocarbons
E907	Refined microcrystalline wax
E920	L-cysteine hydrochloride
E924	Potassium bromate
E925	Chlorine
E926	Chlorine dioxide
E927	Azodicarbonamide (**Azoformamide**)

Haemorrhoids

What are haemorrhoids?

Haemorrhoids or piles are varicosities of the anal canal. In patients with haemorrhoids, the rectal veins have, through prolonged pressure or the ageing process, lost their normal elastic anchoring system within the anal mucosa. The result is obvious dilatation of the veins progressing to prolapse and perianal haematomas. Pain, irritation, exudation including bleeding, and pruritus ani (anal itch) are accompanying symptoms.

Which other clinical conditions can lead to symptoms seen with haemorrhoids?

Bleeding, particularly if profuse and dark, may signal more serious pathology including rectal carcinoma, ulcerative colitis and Crohn's disease. Pruritus ani, which may mimic symptoms of haemorrhoids, is a feature of a variety of problems including threadworm infestations, tinea cruris, scabies, pubic lice infestation and bacterial infections. Careful questioning of patients to identify associated symptoms, and attention to the age of the patients, may help to narrow down the likely possibilities. Thus bleeding without pruritus and anal symptoms may suggest colonic pathology, particularly if the patient is middle-aged or older and has not previously suffered from piles. In all first-time cases referral for a thorough physical examination is recommended. Abdominal pain, vomiting and signs of intestinal obstruction such as indigestion of sudden onset would need urgent attention.

How should haemorrhoids be managed?

Careful evaluation of published data suggests that most cases of haemorrhoids can be managed conservatively by adjustment of diet and local therapy. Only when these fail is surgery required. Initial management of haemorrhoids involves control of symptoms. Regular frequent cleansing of the anal area with soap and warm water will give relief from pruritus ani. A topical anaesthetic may be helpful when irritation becomes unbearable but prolonged application should be avoided because of potential sensitization problems. Actions aimed at providing immediate symptomatic relief should be coupled with measures which will, in the longer term, obviate the need for therapy. Dieting will reduce pressure on the haemorrhoidal veins and change of diet to one with a high fibre content, will minimize straining during defaecation.

What topical remedies are available for the treatment of haemorrhoids?

Astringent formulations containing bismuth salts (e.g. Anusol, Germoloids) are widely used for the control of haemorrhoids, the claimed rationale being that by precipitating proteins the metal ion will form a protective coat. There is little evidence to validate this theory.

Antiseptics such as phenol, chlorhexidine and benzalkonium chloride are included in many anti-haemorrhoidal formulations in the belief that they will prevent secondary infections. Intuitively this appears to be justifiable but there is little published supporting data. Phenol is anaesthetic and anti-pruritic.

Heparinoid, a mucopolysaccharide polysulphate is claimed to possess anti-inflammatory and anti-exudative properties which will of course be useful for the symptomatic control of haemorrhoids. There is a paucity of well-controlled trials to assess heparinoid-containing formulations (e.g. Lasonil) for the management of haemorrhoids.

Rutosides and their derivatives are promoted for the relief of haemorrhoids with the claim that they improve capillary permeability and decrease capillary fragility. The reported positive trials require confirmation.

Shark-liver oil is included in some creams but there is no evidence to show that the oil exerts any benefits additional to those of any other oil used in topical anti-haemorrhoidal formulations.

Precautions and when to refer

(R) Refer when blood not restricted to outside of stool or when bleeding is profuse.

(R) Haemorrhoids associated with marked changes in bowel habit.

(R) Acute episodes which do not improve within a week.

(R) Haemorrhoids accompanied by abdominal symptoms.

Product options

Anaesthetic and/or astringents or emollients
Anacal (heparinoid, laureth 9)
Anodesyn Ointment (lignocaine hydrochloride, allantoin)
Anodesyn Suppositories (lignocaine hydrochloride, allantoin)
Anusol Cream (zinc oxide, bismuth oxide, balsam peru)
Anusol Ointment (zinc oxide, bismuth oxide and subgallate, balsam peru)
Anusol Suppositories (zinc oxide, bismuth oxide, balsam peru)

Germoloids Cream (lignocaine hydrochloride, zinc oxide)
Germoloids Ointment (lignocaine hydrochloride, zinc oxide)
Germoloids Suppositories (lignocaine hydrochloride, zinc oxide)
Hemocane Cream (lignocaine hydrochloride, zinc oxide, benzoic acid, cinnamic acid)
Lanacane Cream (benzocaine, resorcinol, chlorothymol)
Nupercainal Ointment (cinchocaine hydrochloride)
Preparation H Ointment (yeast cell extract, shark liver oil)
Preparation H Suppositories (yeast cell extract, shark liver oil)

Hydrocortisone-containing products

Anusol Plus HC Ointment (hydrocortisone acetate, bismuth oxide and subgallate, benzyl benzoate, balsam peru)
Anusol Plus HC Suppositories (hydrocortisone acetate, zinc oxide, balsam peru, bismuth oxide and subgallate, benzyl benzoate)

Hair loss

What causes hair loss?

Hair loss may have a variety of causes. Fungal infections (tinea capitis), eczema, severe starvation and cytotoxic therapy are examples. However, most commonly hair loss, as seen in balding in males, appears to be due to abnormal reaction of the hair follicles to androgens. Thus application of testosterone to hair follicles from balding scalps leads to further metamorphosis of terminal hair to fine villus hairs probably by shortening the cell cycle of the cells in the hair follicles.

Can hair loss be reversed?

When systemic or skin disease leads to hair loss, recovery to health leads to hair regrowth. Male pattern baldness (alopecia androgenetica) which accompanies ageing is more difficult to reverse. There is no evidence to show that any of the cosmetic or non-prescription hair tonics such as those containing pantothenol and/or cantharides are of any value in male pattern baldness.

Do anti-androgenic drugs work?

Cyproferone acetate and spironolactone are in fact sometimes prescribed for male pattern baldness because of their anti-androgenic effects. Success rates are however low.

Is minoxidil effective?

The evaluation of minoxidil for hair regrowth was initiated because of the serendipitous observation that the antihypertensive drug caused hirsutism as a side-effect. The mechanism for this effect is unknown. Increased perfusion of the hair follicles seems to be an inadequate explanation since local vasodilators are ineffective. The drug has no significant anti-androgenic effects.

The evidence that is available suggests that some bald subjects may benefit from the drug but only as few as one in ten will show hair growth sufficient to make a cosmetic difference. Success appears to be more likely the earlier the drug is applied during the balding process. The affected area should be no larger than 10 mm in diameter and some residual terminal hair should be present at the start of treatment.

Are there any adverse effects of minoxidil?

Little of the topically applied dose is absorbed systemically. Therefore, hypotensive effects are unlikely. Tachycardia, palpitations and non-specific chest pains have been reported occasionally. Inhalation of the sprayed on solution should be minimized. Headache, dizziness and light-headedness have been reported but a causal association with use of minoxidil has not been established. Local irritation, dryness, itching and changes in hair colour have also been reported.

Is minoxidil useful in alopecia areata?

Alopecia areata is a systematic disease which affects both sexes at any age. Typically, patients report a sudden appearance of one or more bald patches. The cause of the baldness is unknown although an autoimmune basis is often suggested. Hair regrows spontaneously in most patients and minoxidil is less useful in this condition than in alopecia androgenica.

Is minoxidil useful in baldness secondary to cytotoxic drug therapy?

With some anticancer drugs, hair loss is essentially a universal side-effect which is reversible on withdrawal of therapy. Minoxidil should not be used for such drug-induced hair loss.

What other precautions should one observe with use of topical minoxidil?

The solution is best applied to the dry scalp. Dyeing and perming of hair are acceptable but sunscreens should be avoided on areas where minoxidil is applied due to possible loss of activity. Head protection is recommended instead. Patients with a history of palpitations, weight gain, oedema, light-headedness or angina should ideally avoid use of minoxidil.

Precations and when to refer

(R) Hair loss in women and children. Cures may lie in treating another complaint.

(R) Sudden onset of hair loss.

(R) Hair loss in individuals who look debilitated as this may indicate systemic disease.

Product options

Regaine Topical Solution (minoxidil)

Halitosis

What causes bad breath and how can it be treated?

Under normal conditions and with proper oral hygiene, human breath is inoffensive. However, bad breath or halitosis may develop for a variety of reasons. These include oropharyngeal or nasal pathology, dental and periodontal problems and ingestion of foods or drugs which lead to odoriferous metabolites excreted through the lungs. An unpleasant breath on awakening is normal as even following proper tooth-brushing sufficient cellular debris accumulates for bacterial proliferation to take place during the night. Since salivary flow and normal swallowing slow down sharply during the night, any odoriferous compounds formed accumulate in the buccal cavity. However, such physiological halitosis readily disappears with the early morning tooth-brushing and oral hygiene. Certain systemic diseases such as uraemia, liver problems and diabetes are also known to be associated with characteristic breaths and indeed in some eastern societies, smelling the breath is still part of the process of clinical investigation.

Management of halitosis will therefore depend on the cause. In many, periodontal treatment and more attention to oral hygiene leads to resolution of the problem but a return to poor oral hygiene may make any improvement only transient. In one recent study of patients troubled with smells, a psychological basis was unveiled in the majority of subjects and corroboration of the subject's complaint is necessary prior to treatment. Reassurance of referral may be all that is required. Foods such as onions and garlic should clearly be avoided when bad breath will offend, although there is now wider acceptance of such items and, by implication, of their adverse effects.

Drugs reported to cause bad breath include disulfiram, isosorbide and topically applied dimethyl sulphoxide. When such drugs are implicated, in practice little can be done except for instituting alternative therapy. Where a microbial origin is suspected, unless acute lesions are observed, antibiotic or long-term antiseptic treatment is not usually advisable because of possible interference with the normal resident flora. Improved oral hygiene should be recommended instead, supplemented if necessary by short-term antiseptic rinses or gels.

See also table under mouth-ulcers.

Precautions and when to refer

 If problem is persistent.

 Halitosis associated with sinus problems.

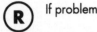 Overuse of mouthwashes and sprays may lead to buccal problems. Phenol-containing products should be used sparingly.

Product options

Betadine Mouthwash (povidone iodine)
Bocasan Mouthwash (sodium perborate)
Chlorhex 2000 Mouthwash (chlorhexidine gluconate)
Corsodyl Mouthwash (chlorhexidine gluconate)
Corsodyl Oral Spray (chlorhexidine gluconate)

Eludril Mouthwash (chlorbutol, chlorhexidine gluconate)
Eludril Spray (chlorhexidine gluconate)
Merocet Mouthwash (cetylpyridinium chloride)
Oraldene Mouthwash (hexetidine)
TCP Liquid Antiseptic (phenol and halogenated phenols)

Standard non-proprietary product
Hydrogen peroxide mouthwash DPF

Hangovers

How does alcohol induce hangovers?

The euphoric feelings which accompany the initial phase of alcohol intoxication are followed by the hangover state, which is characterized by unpleasant mood changes, gastric irritation, lassitude, drowsiness, sleep disturbances, sweating and thirst. The pathogenesis of these symptoms is still poorly defined, although gastric-irritation is widely attributed to a direct irritant effect of the stomach lining by alcohol. Thirst is thought to be due to the mild diuretic effect of alcohol but most of the other symptoms are now no longer thought to be due to metabolic changes. Indeed some studies have shown that despite the biochemical changes seen during the hangover period, including rises in blood levels of lactate, free fatty acid, triglyceride and ketone bodies there is no correlation between these changes and intensity of the hangover. During the hangover stage, which is more intense 12 to 14 hours after initiation of drinking, most of the ethanol and acetaldehyde would have been eliminated from the body.

Current theory suggests that most hangover symptoms are attributable to persistent pharmacological actions of alcohol or its metabolites on the central nervous system and on disturbed hormonal homeostatis.

How should alcohol hangovers be managed?

Advice to avoid further indulgence is unlikely to be heeded. Various non-prescription products are available for alleviating specific symptoms of the hangover syndrome. Paracetamol-based alkaline formulations are helpful in relieving gastric distress and headache. Antacids will relieve gastric irritation when it occurs in isolation from other symptoms. Aspirin-based formulations and ibuprofen are best avoided, although more potent inhibitors of peripheral prostaglandin synthetase have been claimed, with little evidence, to have a prophylactic effect against hangover symptoms. Glucose and fructose may inhibit the metabolic disturbances induced by ethanol but do not affect the symptoms and signs of alcohol intoxication and hangover. Whether sympathy and empathy are justifiable will to a large extent no doubt depend on which church you go to.

Precautions and when to refer

(R) Cases of chronic alcohol abuse.

(R) Patients with abnormal vomit.

(!) Avoid aspirin and ibuprofen-containing formulations as these may exacerbate gastric distress.

(!) Recommend avoidance of tasks requiring complete mental dexterity (e.g. air-piloting, speed driving, etc.) for the next 24 hours as hangovers persist for over 15 hours.

Product options

See under Analgesics (oral).

Hay-fever

What is hay-fever?

Hay-fever is an allergy to pollen grains. Symptoms of the disease are caused by the release of bioactive compounds from mast cells, as the pollen–derived antigens react with the IgE antibody on the surface of the cells. The chemical mediators involved include histamine, prostaglandins, slow reacting substance of anaphylaxis, platelet activation factor and eosinophil chemotactic factor (Figure 7). All these participate in producing the characteristic symptoms of hay-fever, namely, sneezing, rhinorrhoea, congestion, watery eyes and occasionally wheezing and coughing.

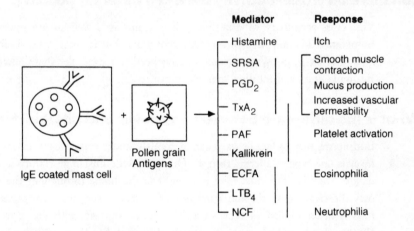

	Mediator	Response
	Histamine	Itch
	SRSA	Smooth muscle contraction
	PGD_2	Mucus production
	TxA_2	Increased vascular permeability
	PAF	Platelet activation
	Kallikrein	
	ECFA	Eosinophilia
	LTB_4	
	NCF	Neutrophilia

SRSA	slow reacting substance of anaphylaxis
PGD_2	Prostaglandin D_2
TxA_2	Thromboxane A_2
PAF	Platelet activating factor
ECFA	Eosinophil chemotactic factor of anaphylaxis
LTB_4	Leukotriene B_4
NCF	Neutrophil chemotactic factor

Fig. 7 Interaction between pollen grain antigens and primed mast cells.

How common is hay-fever?

In a recent study in England and Wales, a prevalence of 20 people per 1000 population was reported for 1981–1982. A cumulative prevalence of symptomatic hay-fever of 10% has been quoted in the literature.

Do all types of pollen cause hay-fever?

The answer is, potentially yes. However, certain types of pollen grains are particularly allergenic. Examples are grass pollen and ragweed pollen. Conifer pollen on the other hand rarely causes rhinitis.

Can one be cured of hay-fever?

The disease tends to resolve itself with age. The first episode usually occurs in childhood or in the teens, depending on exposure intensity and environmental conditions. The condition then tends to worsen for the first two to three seasons before stabilizing and then gradually improving. Desensitization programmes may speed up the resolution of the disease but because this form of therapy may be dangerous and is tedious, it is now less often used. Generally, therefore, hay-fever is treated symptomatically.

Can there be cross-reactivity between different pollens?

Yes, cross-sensitivity to different pollen grains is a well-known phenomenon. Sometimes this may involve very different plants but in some cases similar plants do not cross-react. Water melon and ragweed, for example, share allergens but Bermuda grass and meadow grasses do not.

What is the difference between hay-fever and allergic rhinitis?

Both terms may in fact be used synonymously under certain circumstances. Hay-fever is one type of allergic rhinitis. Others include dust-mite rhinitis and animal dander rhinitis. The dust-mite is present in the home throughout the year and may therefore cause chronic symptoms. For this reason, the term perennial rhinitis is often applied to such an allergy. This contrasts with the term seasonal allergic rhinitis which more accurately describes hay-fever. When there is no obvious cause for the rhinitis, the term vasomotor rhinitis is often used. Underactivity of the sympathetic nervous system and overactivity of the parasympathetic nervous system have been postulated as possible mechanisms for vasomotor rhinitis.

Why are pulmonary symptoms rarely seen in hay-fever?

In hay-fever the allergens are derived from pollen grains. Since pollen grains range in size from about 10 to 100 μm, all are essentially filtered off by the nose. Hence, only the nasal mucosa is exposed to the allergens and the lungs are not normally affected. Only particles smaller than about 5 μm reach the lower respiratory tract. Variability in the biochemical reactivities of lung and nasal tissues may also, of course, contribute to the rarity of pulmonary symptoms, relative to nasal symptoms, in hay-fever.

What other conditions can mimic symptoms of hay-fever?

The common cold, upper respiratory infections in general, perennial rhinitis and vasomotor rhinitis all have common symptoms. A careful history will soon identify cases of true hay-fever. Seasonal patterns in symptoms coinciding with pollen grain shedding strongly suggest hay-fever and the presence of fever would indicate an infective aetiology. Long time hay-fever sufferers will of course readily self-diagnose their own condition. Note that some drugs such as methyldopa, an a receptor antagonist, may cause nasal congestion, while non-selective b antagonists such as propranolol may produce rhinorrhoea.

When are symptoms worst?

Symptoms become worse, the higher the pollen count. Counts are usually high when the weather is dry and breezy. Symptoms of hay-fever also show diurnal variation, often being worst in the early morning.

Why is it that in school children, hay-fever always seems worst at examination time?

There are several possible explanations for this observation. In the United Kingdom, examinations are normally held in the summer months usually at the peak of the pollen season. Hence the severity of symptoms can be expected to be at its height too. It is also well known that the sensitivity of the nose to the allergens increases with the length of exposure, a phenomenon described as 'priming of the end organ'. Hence, intense symptoms coinciding with the height of summer can be expected. Stress is known to exacerbate nasal symptoms in hay-fever patients. Therefore a worsening of symptoms at examination time is not surprising.

Do symptoms of hay-fever show cyclical variations related to the menstrual period?

The available data are very confusing. Some authors have shown no changes in airway responsiveness during the menstrual cycle while others have recommended specific treatments for symptoms of hay-fever showing marked cyclical variations. A systematic study on female hay-fever patients rather than asthmatic patients is required to shed further light on this problem.

What are the available remedies for hay-fever?

Remedies for hay-fever include desensitization, antihistamines and decongestants. H_1 antihistamines (Table 14) are by far the most effective and widely used agents for alleviating the symptoms of hay-fever. Sodium cromoglycate exerts a prophylactic effect, partly by stabilizing mast cells. The antihistamines often fail to relieve nasal congestion and for this reason, decongestants alone or in combination are often used in hay-fever. Desensitization may overcome the underlying allergy

Table 14 Antihistamines in current use in the UK.

Acrivastine	New non-sedative antihistamine – POM
Astemizole	Non-sedative, long-active, slow-acting
Brompheriramine	
Cetirizine	New non-sedative antihistamine
Chlorpheniramine	
Cinnarizine	Used as an anti-motion sickness remedy
Clemastine	
Cyclizine	
Cyproheptadine	One used as an appetite stimulant Significant 5-HT antagonist activity
Dimenhydrinate	Diphenhydramine theophyllinate
Diphenhydramine	
Diphenylpyraline	
Hydroxyzine	Pruritus, short-term anxiety
Loratadine	New non-sedative antihistamine
Mequitazine	POM
Oxatomide	POM
Phenindamine	
Pheniramine	
Promethazine	Used as a sleep aid
Terfenadine	Non-sedative antihistamine
Trimeprazine	POM
Triprolidine	

POM: Prescription Only Medicine

but the occasional serious toxicity remains a problem. In the more severe cases, intranasal steroids are used with more success than with the other commonly used remedies.

Are antihistamine-sympathomimetic eye drops of value for the symptomatic relief of hay-fever?

Eye symptoms are often the most annoying features of hay-fever and antihistamine-decongestant eye drops are often claimed to be effective in providing relief. However, indiscriminate use may lead to elevation of intraocular pressure with possible precipitation of angle closure glaucoma. Occular infections may also be masked and delayed healing has been suggested. These potential dangers have led to the suggestion that all sympathomimetic eye drops should be restricted to prescription only use.

If sympathomimetic drops are not suitable, what else can be recommended?

Sodium cromoglycate eye drops are effective in controlling eye symptoms in hay-fever. A combination of systemic H_1 antihistamine and sodium cromoglycate eye drops is perhaps the best initial therapy for hay-fever patients in whom eye symptoms are severe.

How does desensitization or immunotherapy work?

The precise mechanism of desensitization is still unclear. However, current theory suggests that immunotherapy probably works by stimulating the formation of IgM and IgA antibodies, which act as blocking antibodies to IgE. There is also a shift in the IgG subtypes, from one initially favouring IgG1 to one consisting mainly of IgG4. Reduced basophil reactivity and lymphocyte sensitivity to the allergens, have also been shown after immunotherapy.

Is fexofenadine likely to be safer than terfenadine?

Fexofenadine is the active acid metabolite of terfenadine. It undergoes negligible metabolism and does not appear to cross the blood brain barrier. As the parent compound, it is essentially non-sedative and appears much less likely to interact with other drugs. It should therefore be safer than terfendadine and indeed the Food and Drug Administration has announced its intention to remove products containing terfenadine from the US market now that fexofenadine is available. In the UK the Medicines Control Agency has also proposed a similar course of action and terfenadine will no doubt revert back to prescription only status in due course.

Which antihistamine should one then recommend for hay-fever?

There is insufficient data to compare the toxicity profiles of most of the commonly used antihistamines. Clearly antihistamines such as methapyrilene and mebhy-drolin should be avoided given the wide selection of antihistamines available. The choice of alternatives then essentially depends on relative likelihood of inducing drowsiness and duration of action. The non-sedative cetirizine and loratadine are obvious choices when drowsiness is undesirable. Azatadine and chlorpheniramine are relatively non-sedating. Promethazine and diphenhydramine are among the most sedating and may be the best choice for the control of nocturnal symptoms. Sustained release formulations of chlorpheniramine and brompheniramine increase patient convenience but not necessarily therapeutic profile. Ceterizine has little anticholinergic activity and would therefore be appropriate when the patient already has problems with voiding of the bladder, dry mouth or sexual impotence.

Is it true that hay-fever is more common in patients with other allergies?

This is indeed the case. Allergic diseases are often associated with each other. Thus asthma, hyperplastic sinusitis, hay-fever and eczema often occur concurrently in susceptible patients. Aspirin sensitivity is also often observed in these same patients, although many authorities maintain that exaggerated reactions to aspirin are not immunological in nature.

Are combinations of antihistamines and decongestants useful in hay-fever?

Drug combinations are generally to be avoided in therapy. However, in the case of hay-fever, combinations of antihistamines and decongestants may be worthwhile. Antihistamines on their own often do not relieve the congestion felt by hay-fever sufferers. The sympathomimetic decongestants may also help to counteract the sedative effects of antihistamine compounds. These advantages are, however, counter-balanced by the greater potential for adverse reactions and interactions.

Are there any special risks associated with the use of the newer 'non-sedative' antihistamines?

Although the newer antihistamines, recently donw-regulated as pharmacy-only products, are essentially non-sedative, susceptible individuals can still be affected. More importantly, the ingestion of terfenadine and astemizole recently has been associated with arrythmia. Usually the affected patients have taken higher than the recommended doses or have taken concomitantly drugs which inhibit hepatic metabolism (ketoconazole, itraconazole, erythromycin and other macrolides). Liver dysfunction would be clearly a risk factor too.

Therefore as a safety precaution, patients should not be given terfenadine or astemizole if they:

- are receiving drugs which inhibit hepatic metabolism (ketoconazole, itraconazole, erythromycin, quinine and other macrolide antibiotics and imidazole antifungal drugs);
- suffer from liver diseases;
- drink heavily;
- have a history of arrythmia and other cardiac problems;
- are suffering from thyrotoxicosis;
- may be suffering from electrolyte imbalance (severe diarrhoea or receiving diuretics);
- are taking drugs with arrhythmogenic potential (e.g. antiarrhythmics, neuroleptics, tricyclic antidepressants).

Patients should be referred if they develop signs of arrythmia (palpitations).

Precautions and when to refer

(R) Refer cases not responding to antihistamines.

(!) Interaction between diphenhydramine and other CNS depressants such as temazepam has been reported to lead to perinatal mortality.

(!) Drowsiness common, except for terfenadine and astemizole.

(!) Avoid use of nasal decongestants for hay-fever as chronic use is not recommended – ciliotoxicity.

(!) Avoid antihistamines except chlorpheniramine, cyclizine in acute porphyria.

Product options

Azatadine Tablets (optimine)
Calimal Tablets (chorpheniramine maleate)
Daneral SA Tablets (pheniramine maleate)
Dimotane Tablets (brompheniramine)
Dimotane Elixir (brompheniramine)
Dimotaine LA Tablets (brompheniramine)
Periactin Tablets (cyproheptadine)

Phenergan Tablets (promethazine hydrochloride)
Piriton Syrup (chlorpheniramine maleate)
Piriton Tablets (chlorpheniramine maleate)
Tavegil Tablets (clemastine)
Tavegil Elixir (clemastine)
Thephorin Tablets (phenindamine)

Non-drowsiness-inducing products
Clarityn Syrup (loratadine)
Clarityn Tablets (loratadine)

Zirtek Tablets (cetirizine dihydrochloride)

Steroid-containing products
Beconase Hayfever Spray (beclomethasone dipropionate)

Syntaris Hayfever Nasal Spray (flunisolide)

Second-line agents
Aller-eze Clear Tablets (terfenadine 60 mg)
Hismanal Tablets (astemizole)
Pollon-eze (astemizole)
Seldane (terfenadine)
Terfenor Tablets (terfenadine)

Terflex Tablets (terfenadine)
Terfinax Tablets (terfenadine)
Triludan Tablets (terfenadine)
Triludan Forte Tablets (terfenadine)

Decongestant-containing combinations
Aller-eze Plus Tablets (phenylpropanolamine, clemastine fumarate)
Haymine Tablets (ephedrine hydrochloride, chlorpheniramine maleate)
Resiston-One Spray (xylometazoline, sodium chromoglycate)

Allergic conjunctivitis products
Clariteyes (sodium chromoglycate)
Hay-crom Hay Fever Eye Drops (sodium chromoglycate)
Opticrom Allergy Eye Drops (sodium chromoglycate)
Optrex Hayfever Allergy Eye Drops (sodium chromoglycate)

Headache

What causes headache?

Headache is often subdivided into three main groups according to the mechanism involved: tension headache, produced by muscle contraction or spasm and fatigue, vascular headache, produced by disturbances in normal motor activities of the cranial arteries (e.g. some types of migraine headache – see section on migraine), and traction or inflammation headache, produced by increased pressure on pain-sensitive structures inside or outside the skull (e.g. meningitis, tumour formation and haematoma).

Despite the apparent elegance of the classification, the evaluation of headache and its treatment is extremely difficult. Most headaches respond to non-prescription analgesics. However, it is very important that severe headaches be referred because of their potential seriousness. For example, a sudden agonizing headache is the most common symptom associated with aneurysmal minor bleeds and early detection may reduce the morbidity associated with subarachnoid haemorrhage quite markedly. Even general practitioners often fail to recognise the potential seriousness of such headaches. Other instances for referral are listed below.

Precautions and when to refer

(R) Patients with persistent severe headache.

(R) Headache of severity not previously experienced by patient.

(R) Headache in young children.

(R) Headache associated with head injury.

(R) Headache across the back of head.

(R) Headache with neck stiffness.

(R) Headache associated with visual disturbances.

(R) Headache originating from the temples in older patients (temporal arteritis)

See under migraine also.

See under analgesics.

Product options

See under analgesics and migraine.

Homeopathy

What is homeopathy?

Homeopathy is an approach to therapeutics first proposed by Samuel Hahnemann, a German physician, some 200 years ago. His basic suggestion was that a therapy which produced symptoms resembling those of a disease would be effective against that disease. By careful observation of a patient's symptoms, one could match a remedy to the symptoms. Once this has been done, the minimum dose of the remedy could be chosen to minimize the worsening of the symptoms which were observed at the start of treatment, before the disease improved. While dose-titration is also a feature of orthodox chemotherapy, the distinguishing feature with homeopathy is the extremely high dilutions used. Indeed the dilution could be so extreme that the patient may be unlikely to receive a single molecule of the sup-posedly active remedy. Moreover, homeopaths claim that the greater the dilution the more potent the product. Techniques used in the preparation of homeopathic remedies may also appear absurd to conventional clinicians and scientists. Hah-nemann, for example, reported that violent shaking of solutions somehow improved efficacy.

How widely is homeopathy used?

In many countries of Europe, homeopathic remedies are used by over a third of the public. In Britain, perhaps one in ten adults use them and the trend is increasing.

Are homeopathic remedies effective?

In a recent meta-analysis of over one hundred controlled clinical trials, there was evidence that homeopathic remedies performed better than placebo for certain conditions. Moreover, the evidence in favour of homeopathy appears reproducible. However, because the theories proposed for explaining homeopathic effects appear so absurd, judgement has to be suspended.

Homeopaths would claim that this is unfair, but someone once said that if somebody claims that there is a horse in your neighbour's back-yard, you would find no reason for disbelieving him. However, if the claim were for a unicorn, then you would understandably require much harder evidence.

What are homeopathic potencies?

Potencies are homeopathic preparations with their strengths expressed in terms of dilutions.

X or D refers to 1 in 10 dilutions. Potency described as 3x refers to one prepared by diluting the source material 3 times with a dilution factor 1 in 10 (i.e. $\frac{1}{10} \times \frac{1}{10} \times \frac{1}{10}$ or 10^{-3}).

C refers to 1 in 100 dilutions. Therefore a product labelled 4C has been diluted to 10^{-8} of the original concentration.

M refers to 1 in 1000 dilutions (10^{-3}).

CM refers to one hundred $\frac{1}{1000}$ dilutions.

Recall that Avogadro's number is (6×10^{23}). Therefore, a molar solution diluted to a 12C potency would, on average, contain less than one molecule per litre.

Indigestion

What is indigestion?

Indigestion is the term commonly used by patients to describe vague abdominal discomfort which can be related to meals. One type of indigestion often arises after an abnormal food intake, both in terms of quality and quantity. Binge eating at parties often leads to this type of indigestion which generally resolves itself spontaneously. A second more intractable type is chronic in nature and its aetiological basis is poorly defined and complex.

Common terms used by patients complaining of indigestion include gas, nausea, heartburn, upset stomach, biliousness, gastritis, wind, feeling sick and of course indigestion. Occasionally more impressive terms such as hiatus hernia and dyspepsia are used, probably following a prior encounter with a consultant or other health professional. While some of these terms give a clear indication of a patient's complaint, in most cases further questioning is required before proper advice can be given.

Is dyspepsia a better term to describe the indigestion syndrome described above?

While dyspepsia sounds more sophisticated than indigestion, both terms are probably equally non-descriptive. However, in technical discussions, the term dyspepsia may better convey the fact that a syndrome rather than a specific symptom is being considered.

Can the term hiatus hernia be used interchangeably with dyspepsia?

The oesophagus passes through an opening in the diaphragm, the oesophageal hiatus. In the presence of functional or anatomic abnormality of the oesophageal hiatus, the stomach and other organs may protrude into the thoracic cavity. If this happens, symptoms of gastro-oesophageal distress become evident. Hiatus hernia therefore refers to a distinct anatomical abnormality whereas dyspepsia refers to a syndrome which may of course be observed in the presence of a hiatus hernia.

With hiatus hernia, the most distinct symptoms are those of gastro-oesophageal reflux. Indeed, at one time, the patient with restrosternal discomfort, heartburn and waterbrash was said to suffer from hiatus hernia rather than from today's preferred diagnosis of gastro-oesophageal reflux. Hiatus hernia should therefore ideally be a radiological diagnosis while dyspepsia is essentially a clinical diagnosis. Gastro-oesophageal reflux is often a clinical diagnosis too but intra-oesophageal pH monitoring offers the only definitive diagnostic procedure, although gamma-scintigraphic studies are becoming increasingly used.

Does dyspepsia precede gastro-intestinal ulcers or is it a syndrome associated with the ulcers?

The answer is probably both. Close to half of all patients with classical symptoms of duodenal ulcer show only gastro-duodenal inflammation rather than ulcers but patients with ulcers continue to suffer from dyspepsia. A significant proportion of patients with dyspepsia eventually develop peptic ulcers. Those patients are described as having ulcer dypepsia. In the absence of ulcers and when no under-lying cause can be identified the term non-ulcer dyspepsia or functional dyspepsia is used.

What causes dyspepsia?

Ulceration and gastric or duodenal inflammation have already been referred to. Acid hypersecretion has been shown in some cases but not in others and control of acid secretion does not always give symptomatic relief. Aerophagia, oesophageal or pyloroduodenal dysfunction and the irritable-bowel syndrome, itself a poorly understood entity, have also been put forward as possible causes of dyspepsia. Gastric cancer is a rare cause of dyspepsia. Stress is generally thought to be a possible cause of gastro-intestinal problems leading to dyspepsia.

Various food constituents alter gastro-intestinal mobility and are potentially irritant to the gastro-intestinal mucosa. These foods may therefore induce symptoms of dyspepsia. Tobacco, coffee and alcohol are widely held as being gastric irritants, often by the sufferers themselves. Non-steroidal anti-inflammatory agents often inflict damage to the gastro-intestinal tract and may hence cause dyspepsia. Of the non-prescription drugs, aspirin and ibuprofen are the most significant. Much evidence now shows that *Helicobacter pylori* is a pathogenic organism which invades the gastric mucosa to cause ulcers and symptoms of dyspepsia.

What is the treatment of choice for dyspepsia?

When a potential aetiological factor, such as smoking, excessive stress, irregular meals, alcohol and muco-toxic drugs, can be identified, its removal is the first logical step. Antacids still form the mainstay for the relief of symptoms of dyspepsia on a non-prescription basis. Antacids are also widely prescribed, although histamine H_2 antagonists such as cimetidine, ranitidine and famotidine are now equally widely used. While the results obtained with both H_2 antihistamine and antacids in ulcer-dyspepsia are good, in non-ulcer dyspepsia disappointing outcomes have been reported. Figure 8 shows the site of action of the different types of drugs used in dyspepsia and gastro-intestinal ulcers in general.

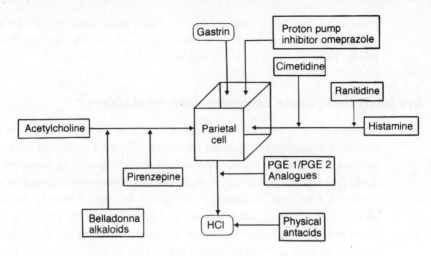

Fig. 8   Effect of neurotransmitters and various agents on acid secretions.

What is gastro-oesophageal reflux?

Gastro-oesophageal reflux, as the name suggests, refers to the regurgitation of the gastric contents into the oesophagus. The acid contents are irritant and therefore the oesophagus develops inflammation and damage (oesophagitis).

How should gastro-oesophageal reflux be managed?

Antacids and antihistamines (H$_2$) are useful for reducing the irritancy of the acid contents. So-called gastric acid reflux suppressants such as the alginate-based formulations (e.g. Gaviscon, Algicon) may help to reduce reflux. Generally, however, dietary management and adoption of appropriate posture are often more useful. Small meals, avoidance of caffeine-containing drinks, missing the last meal, sleeping with the head slightly raised and avoidance of abrupt stooping are all useful measures.

Are mucolytics contraindicated in patients with dyspepsia?

Mucolytics reduce the viscosity of tracheo-bronchial secretions and are therefore commonly used to loosen mucus. Among the mucolytics in clinical use are N-acetyl cysteine, S-carboxymethyl cysteine and bromhexine. In the stomach, mucus provides a protective barrier against autodigestion of gastric tissues by acid. Since mucus from both the respiratory tract and the gastro-intestinal tract contain glyco-proteins, there is the theoretical risk that the mucolytic agents can exert an adverse effect on the gastric mucosa. Indeed, there have been reports of gastric discomfort after oral administration of the mucolytics. Animal experiments also show that the mucolytics decrease mucus thickness and reduce the pH gradient across the mucosal wall. In humans, the levels of N-acetyl muramic acid do not seem to be reduced by S-carboxymethyl cysteine but this may be an inappropriate test for the integrity of the gastric mucosal barrier. Until more positive evidence becomes available it seems wise to withhold mucolytics from patients suffering from gastric ulcers. The contraindication in dyspepsia is much less strong.

Are bacteria a cause of gastro-intestinal ulcers?

Animal experiments have shown that bacteria play an important role in the formation and aggravation of intestinal ulcers induced by irritants such as indomethacin. At one time, it was widely held that the gastric environment was too acidic for bacterial growth until it was shown that *Pseudomonas aeruginosa* could be recovered from most specimens of the gastric mucosa of patients with a gastric ulcer. The pathogenic role of *Helicobacter pylori* (previously known as *Campylobacter pylori*, a spiral organism similar to that identified in the gastric mucosa by Salomon as early as 1896) in causing peptic ulceration is now beyond doubt.

How can acid secretion in the stomach be controlled?

Acid secretion by the parietal cell is stimulated by (1) acetylcholine from the post-ganglionic endings of the vagus nerve, (2) histamine from the mast cells within the gastric mucosa and (3) gastrin from the epithelial cells in the gastric antrum. Potentially therefore, blocking any of the three types of receptors should reduce acid secretion. The evidence that this is indeed the case is provided by the great success of the histamine H_2 inhibitors such as ranitidine and cimetidine. Atropine, a muscarinic blocker, decreases acid secretion but its poor selectivity for the gastric cholinergic receptors leads to unacceptable adverse effects on the heart, vision, urinary system and exocrine glands. Improved selectivity is achieved by agents such as pirenzepine and published data show that this is a viable approach for controlling acid secretion. Effective gastrin receptor blockers are yet to be found, although physical antacids inactivate pepsin by the elevation of gastric pH.

How can antacids interact with concomitantly administered drugs?

Several distinct mechanisms may be involved including:

(1) alteration in ionization of the drug moiety in the gastro-intestinal tract leading to changes in dissolution, partitioning and solubility; this is clearly of significance only for weak electrolytes (e.g. basic antihistamines, non-steroidal anti-inflammatory carboxylic acids);
(2) adsorption of drugs onto insoluble antacids (e.g. digoxin, steroids);
(3) formation of non-absorbable or poorly absorbable complexes (e.g. tetracylines);
(4) altered gastric emptying or gastro-intestinal transit; and
(5) altered disposition by pH-induced changes in urinary excretion (e.g. weak electrolytes such as NSAIDs).

Do corticosteroids cause peptic problems?

High doses of corticosteroids readily produce gastric ulcers in rats, thus suggesting that corticosteroids may be ulcerogenic in humans too. A recent reanalysis of published data showed a significant increase in ulcers in steroid-treated patients relative to controls. Gastro-intestinal haemorrhage was also seen more often in the steroid group. Based on the published data it therefore appears that there may be a link between corticosteroid therapy and peptic ulceration but the link is only marginal. Patients with a previous ulcer or with diseases predisposing to peptic ulceration (e.g. rheumatoid arthritis, hepatic cirrhosis) should therefore avoid corticosteroids.

Can antacid therapy predispose to infections?

This is indeed an interesting possibility. The normally low pH of the stomach provides a formidable barrier against the ingress of bacteria in ingested food, although *Helicobacter pylori* seems to be an exception. Therefore, theoretically, an increase in pH may reduce the integrity of this gastric barrier. Indeed studies with omeprazole show that when acid secretion is decreased substantially, then bacterial count and nitrate and N-nitrosamine concentrations in gastric juice increase. Typhoid bacilli present a particular risk and the Brucella species has given cause for concern. Therefore, it has been suggested that antacids should perhaps not be given when the risk of exposure to brucellosis and enteric fever is high, such as during travel to areas where these infective organisms are endemic.

Which is the best antacid?

There is no unique answer to this question as the indication considered will affect the final choice. Ideally an antacid should produce rapid acid neutralization and yet exert a sustained activity. It should be free of adverse effects and palatable but should not be excessively expensive. None of the available antacids is ideal and combinations of antacids are often used to improve the activity profile of the individual antacid components.

What are non-absorbable antacids?

Antacids such as aluminium hydroxide and magnesium trisilicate were at one time thought not to be absorbed into the systemic circulation; hence the term non-absorbable. Recent data however show that the 'non-absorbable' antacids in fact lead to significant increases in serum metal ions. Serum aluminium concentration, for example, doubles after a 4-week ingestion of near therapeutic doses of aluminium magnesium hydroxides combinations.

How does peppermint oil work as a carminative?

Peppermint oil and essential oils in general, are known to inhibit gastro-intestinal smooth muscle and this may well provide the basis for peppermint oil's mode of action as an antispasmodic and carminative. Recent work suggests that menthol, the main constituent of peppermint oil, may act as a calcium channel inhibitor and products which specifically deliver the oil in the colon are currently widely promoted for the relief of the irritable bowel syndrome.

Do aluminium-containing antacids lead to senile dementia?

Recent work on the prevalence of Alzheimer's, a condition characterized by dementia, shows that there is a correlation between the prevalence of the disease and the aluminium content of water. An association does not however prove causation, but given that there are safer alternatives, aluminium-containing antacids are best avoided.

With the huge success of the histamine H_2 inhibitors, should antacids now be discarded?

It is indeed tempting to suggest that the antacids should now be considered obsolete. However, the available evidence shows that they are very much first-line choices for most non-prescription indications associated with dyspepsia. Indeed, recent controlled trials have demonstrated that they are certainly as good as cimetidine for both treatment and prophylaxis of duodenal ulcers and some authorities are now recommending that in the trial of any new H_2 blocker, antacids should be used as an active control.

Are there any clinically important differences between the H_2 antagonists now available OTC?

The three OTC H_2 antagonists (cimetidine, ranitidine and famotidine) are equally effective in preventing meal-induced symptoms of indigestion and hyperacidity. The only difference is in their potential side-effect profile. Cimetidine inhibits the cytochrome P450 hepatic mixed function oxidase system and binds to androgen receptors. Potentially therefore it is likely to be involved in a wider spectrum of adverse effects and therefore less suitable as an OTC drug. Pharmacists recommending OTC cimetidine should make sure that their patients avoid drugs which are metabolised by the cytochrome P450 system, notably warfarin, theophylline, aminophylline, nifedipine and phenytoin which have narrow therapeutic windows. Others will no doubt come to light from time to time and vigilance is required.

Some studies have suggested that H_2 antagonists interact with alcohol. Is this important?

Reduced clearance of alcohol has been reported to follow concomitant ingestion of H_2 antagonists. However, the evidence has been contradictory and any effects observed has been sufficiently small to suggest no clinically important consequences.

Precautions and when to refer

R Refer patients older than 45 and complaining of severe dyspepsia for the first time (possible malignancy).

R Dyspepsia associated with dark stools (ulceration and perforation).

R Dyspepsia associated with marked weight loss (malignancy).

R Patients vomiting black or bloody material (ulceration or perforation).

R Patients with pain going through the back (heart problems).

R Patients not relieved by antacids (heart problems).

R Children with indigestion not related to excessive food intake.

R Severe pain made worse on effort (angina).

! Avoid aluminium-containing antacids; use magnesium-containing products instead in acute porphyria.

! Avoid ranitidine in acute porphyria.

! Potentially important antacid–drug interactions.

Oral contraceptives	Penicillamine	Quinidine
Chloroquine	Phenothiazines	Tetracyclines
Digoxin	Phenytoin	(multivalent antacids)
Isoniazid	Prednisone	Theophylline
NSAIDs	Procainamide	Valproic acid
Lithium	Pyrimethamine	

! Potential adverse effects.

Agent	Disadvantage
Aluminium hydroxide	Potential accumulation in nerve tissues. Potential increase in calcium excretion. Laxative effect.

Aluminium phosphate	Potential accumulation. Laxative effect. Poor buffer capacity.
Calcium carbonate	Rebound acidity at high doses.
Magnesium carbonate	Hypermagnesaemia at high doses.
Magnesium trisilicate	Poor buffer capacity. Silica content.
Sodium bicarbonate	Sodium content. Short acting.

 General recommendations

For acute indigestion, a calcium or magnesium carbonate antacid usually provides prompt relief.

An H_2 antagonist may help prevent symptoms in those known to be susceptible to indigestion caused by specific foods.

Selected product options

Neutralizing antacids
Andrews Antacid Tablets (calcium and magnesium carbonates)
Gaviscon Liquid (sodium bicarbonate, calcium carbonate and sodium alginate)
Nulacin Tablets (calcium and magnesium carbonates)
Remegel Tablets (calcium carbonate)
Rennie Tablets (calcium and magnesium carbonates)
Setlers Tablets (calcium carbonate)
Tums (calcium carbonate)

H_2 antagonists

Pepcid AC Tablets
(Famotidine)

Tagamet Dual Action
Suspension
(Cimetidine, sodium
alginate)

Zantac Tablets
(Ranitidine)

Ingrown toenails

What causes ingrown toenails and how should they be treated?

Ingrown toenails are caused by pressure to the nails leading to bacterial invasion. Treatment usually involves removing the offending section of the nail followed by antimicrobial drug cover and the subsequent wearing of better shoes. Non-prescription remedies are usually inadequate. Nails should be cut straight across without injuring the underlying nail bed particularly at the edges.

Insect bites and stings

How do insect venom and bites inflict damage to tissues?

With stings, the initial damage is caused by the direct pharmacological activities of the constituents of the venom. Melittin haemolyses, apamin exerts a neurotoxic effect and mast cell degranulating peptides cause the release of histamine. The venom itself may contain histamine, dopamine, noradrenaline, 5-hydroxytryptamine and acetylcholine, all of which are pharmacologically active. These chemical constituents, however, exert only mild local effects from the doses injected by the insects. The more serious damage is the result of allergic reactions to constituents of the venom, in particular phospholipases and hyaluronidase. Each year a few people in fact die as a result of anaphylactic reactions to insect venom. With insect bites, local reactions are due to allergic responses to the secretions of the insects or to their residues. Bullous reactions are occasionally seen but more generally mild erythema, inflammation and intense itchiness are the only signs of the insect bites.

How should insect stings and bites be managed?

Wasps do not leave their stings behind. With bee stings, extraction of the sting is the first step. The quicker the removal, the smaller the weal will be. Application of Calamine lotion is useful, both to alleviate the itch and to produce a cooling effect. Crotamiton may also be useful as an antipruritic agent. Local anaesthetics are disappointing because of poor penetration through the skin.

In patients known to be allergic to insect venom, immediate help is required and an H_1 antihistamine given orally may help reduce subsequent reactions. Patients known to show severe reactions should carry a prescribed insect kit and be shown how to self-inject 0.3 ml of a 1:1000 adrenaline solution. A puff from an adrenaline spray (Medihaler-Epi) may also produce the same beneficial effects and may be an adequate alternative to parenteral adrenaline.

Antiseptic creams or alcohols may help provide cover against secondary infections. There is less rationale for the use of astringents and calcium and vitamin D despite isolated reports of their usefulness.

Should desensitization be recommended?

Desensitization is certainly an effective method but it is not without risk. Strict supervision by a clinical allergist is required. Desensitization is particularly contraindicated in patients developing serum reaction with urticaria, joint pain, fever and lymphadenopathy within 10 days of an insect sting or bite. Desensitization should be carried out with pure venom extracts rather than with whole insect extracts.

Are non-steroidal anti-inflammatory agents (NSAIDs) useful to relieve insect stings?

Theoretically there is a case for using NSAIDs to alleviate the inflammation and pain associated with insect stings. However, there have been reports of exaggerated responses to insect stings in patients on concomitant NSAIDs. Therefore, NSAIDs should not be recommended for the relief of stings until this issue has been clarified.

Are insect repellents worthwhile?

Insect stings and bites are at best a nuisance, but at worst such bites or stings may be fatal. Anaphylactic reactions to insect venom and the transmission of parasitic infections such as malaria, cause most concern. An effective and safe insect repellent is therefore very worthwhile. The most widely used insect repellent is diethyl toluamide (DEET), either alone or in combination with ethohexadiol or ethylhexanediol and dimethyl phthalate (DMP). Some pyrethroids are also being considered as insect repellents.

The long history of use of DEET and DMP shows that these agents are both effective and generally safe when used as recommended by the manufacturers. However, significant amounts of insect repellents are absorbed following application to the skin, and in children toxic reactions leading to fatalities have been reported. Therefore particular care must be exercised with children and with application on broken skin or mucous membrane.

As with any problem with percutaneous absorption, an increase in skin temperature is likely to increase the extent of absorption. Therefore hot baths and saunas should be avoided after application of the insect repellent. Some patients may be sensitive to the insect repellents and a preliminary test over a small area of the skin is advisable. Contact with plastics such as spectacle frames, contact lenses and acetate clothing should be avoided. Products containing concentrations higher than 50% DEET may lead to skin blistering and scar-formation. Oral ingestion may be rapidly fatal.

These problems have led to a call for the withdrawal of products containing more than 75% DEET from general use. Sprays are usually more comfortable to use than sticks or semi-solid formulations and products containing high levels of the repellents are oily and unpleasant to apply.

Precautions and when to refer

 Patients showing signs of severe allergy to insect bites or stings, particularly if respiratory symptoms, wheeziness, fainting or generalized skin rashes are present. All such patients should ideally carry an emergency single-dose adrenaline injector or inhaler with them.

 A dose of antihistamine tablets or syrup is recommended as a precautionary measure, even if symptoms are absent, in patients with a history of severe allergy to insect venom.

Product options

Hydrocortisone-containing cream
Eurax HC Cream (hydrocortisone, crotamiton)

HC45 Cream (hydrocortisone)
Nortisone Cream (hydrocortisone)

Local anaesthetics
Dermidex Cream (lignocaine, chlorbutanol, celrimide, chlorhydroxyallantorinate)
Lanacane Cream (benzocaine)
Solarcane Cream (benzocaine, triclosan)
Solarcane Spray (benzocaine, triclosan)

Wasp-eze Spray (benzocaine, mepyramine)

Topical antihistamine
Aller-eze Cream (diphenhydramine)
Anthisan Cream (mepyramine)
Caladryl Cream (diphenhydramine, camphor)

Caladryl Lotion (diphenhydramine, camphor)
Histergan (diphenhydramine)
Wasp-eze Cream (antazoline)

Others
Eurax Cream (crotamiton)
Eurax Lotion (crotamiton)
Lacto-calamine Lotion (phenol, witch hazel)

Stingose Spray (aluminium sulphate)
Witch Doctor Stick (witch hazel)

Itch

What causes pruritus?

A whole variety of physical stimuli (e.g. thin wire strokes, heat and cold) and chemical stimuli (e.g. histamine and kinins) evoke the itch sensation. Other substances such as the prostaglandins lower the threshold for the itch response. Substances identified so far as being able to initiate the itch response either directly or indirectly include those shown in Table 15.

Table 15 Substances which may cause itch.

Histamine	Opiod peptides
5-hydroxytryptamine	Prostaglandins (indirectly)
Neuropeptides	PGE_2
Bombesine	PGH_2
Neurotensin	Proteases or endopeptidases
Secretin	Chymotrypsin
Substance P	Kallikrein
Vasoactive intestinal	Papain
peptide (VIP)	Trypsin
Opiates	

How is itch actually caused by these pruritic stimuli?

The mechanisms are complex and the physiological and pathophysiological bases of the itch responses are still subject to much controversy. It is known that itch receptors are free unmyelinated nerve endings associated with the skin, mucous membranes and the cornea. The current majority view is that these receptors are polymodal, although itch is generally regarded as being a primary modality rather than sub-threshold pain. The complexity of it all is exemplified by the fact that low intradermal doses of histamine cause itch while higher doses lead to pain.

A number of substances such as VIP and secretin are thought to cause itch by liberating histamines. Others such as the prostaglandins are thought to potentiate the pruritic effect of other mediators rather than acting directly on the itch receptors. The mechanisms by which other substances such as mucanain, an endopetidase and kallikrein cause itch are still conjectural.

What diseases is itch associated with?

Itch may be a symptom of a variety of diseases (Table 16). Among these are both cutaneous and systemic diseases. Well known examples of skin diseases associated

Table 16   Diseases associated with itch.

Skin and localized diseases or irritation	Systemic diseases
Bullous pemphigoid	Endocrine diseases:
Chemical sensitivities	diabetes
(e.g. washing powders)	thyroid malfunction
Chickenpox	Iron deficiency anaemia
Dermatitis:	Neurological problems
atopic	Obstructive biliary disease:
contact	primary biliary cirrhosis
herpetiformis	intrahepatic cholestasis
Dermatophytic infections:	of pregnancy
athlete's foot	Oncological disease:
ringworm	carcinoma
Fibre glass deposition	Hodgkin's disease
Folliculitis	lymphoma
Hay-fever	mutiple myeloma
Lichen planus	Psychiatric disturbances:
Measles	delusional parasitosis
Miliaria	dermatitis artefacta
Parasitic infestations:	Renal failure (uraemia)
echinococcosis	
onchocerciasis	
pediculosis	
scabies	
trichinosis	
Pruritus ani	
Pruritus vulvae	
Psoriasis	
Sunburn	
Xerosis (dryness)	

with pruritus are parasitic diseases, eczema and pruritus ani. Cholestatic liver disease and a number of haematological diseases are examples of systemic diseases which may have itch as a symptom.

How can one identify the cause of itch?

A careful history of the symptom is essential. In many cases, as with hay fever, the cause is obvious. In others the distribution of the itch gives valuable information and may lead to identification of scabies, pediculosis and pruritus ani or vulvae. The temporal appearance of the itch and itch affecting more than one member of the family may also help in diagnosis. The presence of bed bugs and pet insects may thereby be revealed. Itching behind the knees and at skin folds suggest a dermatitis as does stress-related episodes of pruritus. Aquagenic urticaria characterized by itch after water exposure is also well described. Itch may also be a feature of food intolerance. Wines, fish, nuts, strawberries and food colours are commonly claimed

Table 17   Drugs which may cause itching and other alterations in skin sensation.

Pruritus

Acetohexamide	Melphalan
Amiloride	Methprylone
Amitriptyline	Lanatoside C
Beclamide	Metronidazole
Captopril	Miconazole
Cefadroxil	Nalbuphine
Cefoxitin	Niclosamide
Ceftazidime	Nortriptyline
Ceftizoxime	Phenazocine
Cephazolin	Probenecid
Chloroquine	Procainamide
Chenodeoxycholic acid	Sulindac
Cinoxacin	Sulphasalazine
Diflunisal	Tamoxifen
Doxepin	Thiabendazole
Etretinate	Timolol
Fenoprofen	Tinidazole
Glipizide	Tobramycin
Gold	Triazolam
Hydroxocobalamin	Trimethoprim
Isotretinoin	Vidarabine
Ketoconazole	

Paraesthesia

Acetazolamide	Iproniazid
Allopurinol	Isocarboxazid
Amikacin	Maprotiline
Amiloride	Methyldopa
Amitriptyline	Mexiletine
Benztropine	Nadolol
Captopril	Netilmicin
Ceftazidime	Nortriptyline
Ceftizoxime	Perhexiline
Chlorpropamide	Phenelzine
Cisplatin	Prazosin
Clomipramine	Propranolol
Cycloserine	Sulindac
Cyproheptadine	Sulthiame
Dacarbazine	Timolol
Diflunisal	Tocainide
Doxepin	Viloxazine
Ethambutol	Vinglastine
Guanethidine	Vincristine
Hydrocortisone	

Tingling of skin or scalp

Calcitonin	Dihydroergotamine
Cinoxacin	Labetalol
Dexamethasone	Prednisolone

to cause itching. The presence of blisters suggests more serious diseases like bullous pemphigoid and dermatitis herpetiformis.

Any persistent itch associated with signs of systemic changes (weight loss, fever, gastro-intestinal disturbance and xantholasmata) suggests even more serious diseases which should be excluded. Among these diseases are carcinoma and biliary cirrhosis.

Is itch a potential side-effect of drugs?

Some drugs are indeed known to cause itching as a side-effect. Chloroquine is a well known example. Others are listed in Table 17.

What is the best treatment for pruritus?

If there is an underlying pathology which is leading to the pruritus then clearly specific treatment is the best approach. In the vast majority of cases no specific underlying abnormality can be identified and the itch episodes are transient and self-limiting. Under these circumstances symptomatic treatment is the best approach. H_1 antihistamines given orally are successful in many instances. The nasal and conjunctival itch associated with hay-fever is effectively relieved by antihistamines (H_1). At one time it was thought that only the centrally-active antihistamines suppress itch. It is now known that the peripherally-acting ones may be effective too.

Pruritus ani and vulvae are best managed by regular cleansing with warm soapy water. Anaesthetic gels may provide additional relief. The itch accompanying viral skin diseases (chickenpox and measles) is relieved by calamine lotion, probably through its phenolic content. Pruritus associated with eczema may respond well to warm water and a moisturizing application such as emulsifying ointment. Hydrocortisone cream may of course be particularly useful here too. More recently the antipruritic properties of crotamiton have been re-emphasized.

Precautions and when to refer_____

 Persistent itch, particularly if associated with weight loss.

 Be alert for drug-induced itch.

Product options _____

Oral antihistamine products (see under
  hay-fever products)
Topical antihistamine products (see under
  insect stings)

Eurax Cream (crotamiton)
Eurax Lotion (crotamiton)

Jet lag

What is jet lag?

Jet lag is the term applied to describe the period of unease which often follows travel across time zones or to different climatic conditions. Classical symptoms, aside from general unease, include loss of appetite, disturbed sleep, suboptimal performance and disorientation.

What causes jet lag?

There is as yet no consensus but one theory is that jet lag is due to desynchronization of normal biorhythms. There has been some suggestion that the disturbed secretion of melatonin by the pineal gland may be responsible for the loss in rhythmicity. Some cynics suggest that jet lag is a mythical problem and if it exists is probably caused by alcohol poisoning and excessive food.

What remedies are available for jet lag?

Melatonin, a hormone produced by the pineal glands of animals, but now synthesized, has been shown to improve subjective feelings in some studies. It is not available currently as a health supplement in the UK but can be bought at airports. Short-acting hypnotics are widely thought to be useful. Mineral water and light meals are promoted by some as being the most rational prophylaxis against jet lag.

Lice

How should a louse infestation be treated?

A suitable pediculicide should be recommended. Lotions are theoretically preferable to shampoos but the latter are more acceptable to patients. Because all of the currently used pediculicides are not completely ovicidal, a second application a week after the first is usually recommended. Children from the same family are usually simultaneously infected. Careful examination of the hair is required and simultaneous treatment initiated if required. In the absence of infestation treatment should be withheld.

Which product should be recommended as prophylaxis against the louse?

None of the parasiticides should be recommended as prophylactic agents. They all have high lipophilicity and readily permeate the skin. Systemic toxicity is therefore a real possibility on repeated applications, particularly since accumulation may occur in the fatty tissues of the body. Resistance may also become an increasing problem with repeated use of the parasiticides.

How many types of lice are there?

Three distinct types of lice are commonly observed in man: the head louse, the body louse and the pubic louse, commonly referred to as the crab louse or 'crabs'. The claw like forelegs of the crab louse give it a distinct appearance from the other lice. The head louse is the most common, affecting well over 100 000 children annually in the United Kingdom. The body louse is usually seen among vagrants, thereby giving the impression that the louse can only affect the unclean individual. The body louse can become devastating at times of population overcrowding such as during wars and following natural disasters.

How are lice transmitted?

Hair to hair or body contact is usually necessary. Indeed, pubic lice are usually transmitted through sexual contact. Although it is said that adults commonly transmit head lice to children, common experience would suggest that the school playground is probably the most effective medium for lice transmission.

What are the most effective pediculicides?

Six parasiticides generally available in the UK for use on humans are carbaryl, crotamiton, dicophane (DDT), gamma benzene hexachloride (lindane), malathion and pyrethrins. Synergized pyrethrins and synthetic pyrethroids are available. Malathion is the preferred pediculicide because of its high efficacy against the parasites. Carbaryl, once a preferred pediculicide, has now been up-regulated to prescription only use because of concerns about its potential carcinogenicity. Naturally-occurring pyrethrins are safe and effective but lack ovicidal activity because of rapid breakdown to inactive compounds. The synthetic pyrethroids, permethrin and phenothrin, are recent introductions. Early results are encouraging but longer term experience is required before sensible comparisons can be made with the better established pediculicides. In particular, attention will need to focus on possible parasitic resistance to them, a problem already quite serious with gamma benzene hexachloride and to a lesser extent with carbaryl and malathion. Rotational use is usually recommended by public health authorities.

An earlier shampoo formulation (Full Marks Shampoo) was withdrawn by the manufacturers because of a number of ocular reactions probably due to the formulation excipients rather than to the phenothrin but an interaction could not be excluded.

Gamma benzene hexachloride (lindane) still has its proponents – but its use is declining because of its long half-life of over 3 months in the human body. Indeed some manufacturers have discontinued lindane – containing anti-louse products and the Food and Drug Administration now regards lindane as a second-line agent. Benzyl benzoate, monosulfiram, crotamiton and dicophane are now relatively rarely used against lice infestations in the UK. Benzyl benzoate and crotamiton have poor activity against the louse while dicophane accumulates in the body and is environmentally damaging.

How serious is the problem of resistance to the pediculicides?

Resistance to the main insecticidal compounds develops rapidly and is the main problem associated with the regular use of these compounds in the community. Indeed because of this problem, it is suggested that use of malathion and carbaryl should be rotated about every 3 years and guides relating to resistance to these two compounds are now reported in the pharmaceutical press at regular intervals.

How do the pediculicides work?

Both malathion and carbaryl are choline esterase inhibitors. In humans, malathion is hydrolysed to the acid forms which are further decomposed by plasma phosphatases before excretion as succinic acid and water-soluble phosphates in the urine. Insects, including the louse, on the other hand activate the drug further to malaoxon and die as a result. Carbaryl is also rapidly detoxified by the human body to 1-naphthol. In insects, this detoxification is much slower, although this may accelerate many-fold in resistant lice. Gamma benzene hexachloride interferes with ion transport across nerve membranes and hence paralyses the insect. The pyrethroids interfere with carbohydrate metabolism within the insects.

Are shampoos better than lotions?

From the point of view of patient acceptance a shampoo is usually preferable to a lotion. In most cases shampoos perform as well as lotions since although dilution of the active agent during shampooing and sequestration by the surfactants lead to decrease in effective concentration, this is made up for by more homogeneous distribution of the agent. However, poorly formulated shampoos may be associated with high failure rates and this had led some authors to recommend lotions in preference to shampoos. One or two repeat applications may be necessary with both formulations. Indeed some authorities recommend two repeats at 3-daily intervals, when shampoos are used. Twelve-hour lotions are generally regarded as more effective than the 2-hour products.

Is prophylactic use of the pediculicides worthwhile?

Prophylaxis is generally not recommended because of the increased risk of resistance and because of potential accumulation of the insecticides following repeated applications.

Should the whole family be treated?

At one time, it was generally recommended that if a member of the family, typically a child, is infected, then the whole family should be treated on a prophylactic basis. This is now no longer the consensus view and indeed we would now recommend the 'wait and see' approach.

What advice should be given to patients using the pediculicides?

(1) The manufacturers' instructions should be followed as closely as possible.
(2) The alcohol-containing lotions are flammable and should be kept away from flames, as should the treated hair.
(3) Lotions should be applied liberally to ensure complete coverage.
(4) The shampoo may be repeated twice at 3 days' intervals.
(5) The product should not be used prophylactically.
(6) Advice should be sought if any potential user is an epileptic, anorexic, asthmatic or pregnant.

Are louse repellents useful?

Recently louse repellent formulations based on piperonal have been introduced. There is little in-vivo field data to demonstrate their effectiveness. Moreover given that their toxicity and irritancy profiles on long-term application have not been defined, they cannot as yet be recommended.

Precautions and when to refer

(R) If secondary infection present.

(R) If eradication of scabies not successful after two treatments.

(!) Do not use gamma benzene hexachloride in epileptics as the drug accumulates and interferes with nerve conduction.

(!) Do not use gamma benzene hexachloride and dicophane during pregnancy and lactation. Limit use of all insecticides during pregnancy.

(!) Do not use gamma benzene hexachloride in the anorexic and those with very low body weight.

(!) Do not use gamma benzene hexachloride in those under 3 years.

(!) Asthmatics may develop attacks when exposed to insecticides.

Product options

Derbac-M Liquid (malathion)
Full Marks Lotion (phenothrin)
Lyclear Cream Rinse (permethrin)
Prioderm Shampoo (malathion)

Quellada M Lotion (malathion)
Quellada M Shampoo (malathion)
Suleo M Lotion (malathion)

Second-line products for lice
Ascabiol Emulsion (benyl benzoate)

Products recently up-regulated to prescription only status
Carylderm Lotion (carbaryl)
Clinicide Lotion (carbaryl)

Derbac C Lotion (carbaryl)
Suleo C Lotion (carbaryl)

Products now withdrawn
Quellada Lotion (lindane/gamma benzene hexachloride)

Malaria

What is malaria?

Malaria is an infection caused by parasites of the genus *Plasmodium*. Four species of the parasite are known to cause human infection – *Plasmodium vivax*, *Plasmodium ovale*, *Plasmodium malariae* and *Plasmodium falciparum*. Symptoms of the disease show characteristic periodicity and include fever, nausea, shivers and in the case of falciparum malaria, convulsions.

How common is malaria in Britain?

Although malaria is no longer endemic in Britain, the massive increases in international travel to and from malarious areas mean that there is a significant number of patients with malaria in Britain. A survey covering the period 1977–1986 indicates a steady increase in the number of cases over the past few years. In 1986, over 2300 cases were reported and *P. falciparum* accounted for about a third of those cases. Four deaths were reported in the same year. The vast majority of *P. falciparum* malaria cases were from Africa. The Indian subcontinent contributed more of the *P. vivax* cases (640 cases in 1986) but few of the *P. falciparum* cases (35 cases in 1986). About a third of all malaria cases reported in Britain were in immigrants visiting friends or relatives in their countries of origin. Foreign visitors and new immigrants together account for about a further third of all cases.

How is malaria acquired?

Malaria is usually acquired through mosquito bites. Injection of the sporozoites into the skin of the human victim, by the infected mosquito, is followed by systemic dissemination and deposition of the parasites in the liver. The hepatocyte acts as a development site for the parasite. The mature schizonts rupture to liberate merozoites into the circulation. These then parasitize erythrocytes and undergo asexual schizogony. Except for *Plasmodium malariae* schizonts which take 72 hours to develop, the erythrocytic schizonts take 48 hours to mature. Upon maturation, the schizonts lead to rupture of the host cells and the characteristic periodic nature of the symptoms. Some merozoites develop into sexual forms known as gametocytes and these infect other mosquitoes to perpetuate the infection cycle.

Why is falciparum malaria particularly severe?

Symptoms of malaria are caused by reduction in flexibility and increased adhesiveness of the parasitized erythrocytes. This in turn leads to capillary occlusion, kinin activation, increased capillary permeability and the deposition of immune complexes. The severity of the symptoms is obviously dependent on the parasitic load which tends to be particularly high in falciparum malaria.

Is vaccination likely to be an effective prophylaxis against malaria?

Natural immunity against the malarial parasite is known to develop following repeated infections. However, such immunity is slow to develop and is rarely total. Protection is known to be passively transferable between people and transplacental transfer of protective antibodies from the mother to the foetus is widely accepted. Vaccination therefore appears to be a viable approach for providing prophylaxis against malaria. However, despite much effort by a number of research groups, an effective anti-malarial vaccine remains an elusive goal.

If an effective vaccine is not available what are the possible prophylactic measures against malaria?

Chemoprophylaxis remains the best alternative, although the choice of a suitable drug is not easy, particularly because of the current spread of resistant species of the parasite around the world. *P. vivax*, for example, is now resistant to dihydrofolate reductase inhibitors in some countries and *P. falciparum* is commonly resistant to the 4-aminoquinolines (Table 18). In addition to chemoprophylaxis, visitors to malarious areas may benefit from use of insect repellents (diethyltoluamide sticks or sprays) and from protective nets at night.

Table 18   Classification of drugs which have been used as prophylactics against malaria.

4-aminoquinolines	Amodiaquine
	Chloroquine
Dihydrofolate reductase inhibitors	Proguanil
	Pyrimethamine
	Trimethoprim
Sulphonamides and sulphones	Sulphadoxine
	Dapsone

Table 18 lists some of the drugs which have been used for the prophylaxis of malaria. Recent evidence suggests that amodiaquine and pyrimethamine/sulfadoxine (Fansidar) are too toxic for use as prophylactic agents. Both the combination pyrimethamine/sulfadoxine and amodiaquine have been associated with agranulocytosis and other blood dyscrasias. Given that malaria reference laboratories are now set up in the UK, we recommend that readers check up on the latest advice from these centres. For travel prophylaxis telephone 0171 636 8636. Recorded advice is available for travellers on 0171 388 9600.

When should prophylactic anti-malarial drugs be given?

Effective blood concentrations can be achieved rapidly with recommended dosages. However, it is generally agreed that therapy should start about a week before exposure to the malarious area, in order to accustom the traveller to taking the drug regularly. It is also generally recommended that prophylaxis should be administered for at least 4 weeks after leaving the malarious area in order to ensure that the hepatic phase is adequately covered. Even such lengthy post-exposure prophylaxis may not be adequate for preventing *P. vivax* resurgence. Therefore, all travellers returning from malarious areas should be advised to report unexplained fevers as soon as possible so that infection can be excluded.

Should infants be given chemoprophylaxis against malaria?

Infants born to non-immune mothers have no protection against malaria and should therefore be given chemoprophylaxis when visiting malarious areas. Chloroquine syrup, alone or in combination with proguanil, is usually recommended.

How do the anti-malarial agents work?

The available anti-malarials attack the parasites at various stages of their development. The sites of action are shown in Figure 9. Chloroquine, proguanil and dapsone attack the erythrocytic asexual schizonts. Proguanil also inhibits the hepatic pre-erythrocytic forms.

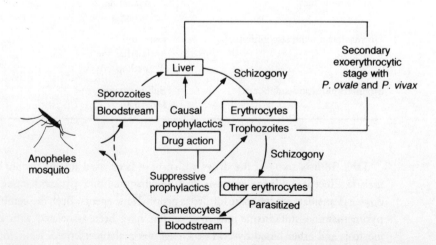

Fig. 9   Life cycle of the malaria parasite and site of action of prophylactic agents.

Is malaria chemoprophylaxis safe during pregnancy?

Exposure to all drugs, including the anti-malarial drugs, should ideally be avoided during pregnancy and the pregnant woman should therefore seriously consider whether visits to a malarious area should be postponed. If postponement is not acceptable, then chemoprophylaxis should be recommended since contracting the disease carries with it serious complications which outweigh the potential risks of exposure to the chemoprophylactic agents. Chloroquine and proguanil are again probably the safer drugs, although ocular and inner ear damage may occur in infants of mothers exposed to high doses of chloroquine, throughout pregnancy. Because of these potential problems, chemoprophylaxis of malaria during pregnancy should not be undertaken on a non-prescription basis.

Table 19   Adverse effects of antimalarial agents.

Amodiaquine	Blood dyscrasias
	Hepatotoxicity
	Pigmentation of nail bed
Chloroquine	Retinal damage at high doses
	Skin itching
	Exacerbation of psoriasis
	Intestinal upsets
Dapsone/pyrimethamine	Agranulocytosis
(Maloprim) POM in UK	Folate deficiency
	Neonatal methaemoglobinaemia
	and haemolysis
Proguanil	Abdominal disturbance
Pyrimethamine	Folate deficiency
	Insomnia at high doses
	Skin rash
Sulphadoxine/pyrimethamine	Severe skin reactions
(Fansidar) POM in UK	notably Steven-Johnson Syndrome
	Bone marrow depression
	Agranulocytosis

Is it true that some plants are effective against malaria?

This is certainly true. Quinine, the cinchona alkaloid is still useful in the management of malaria and some authorities indeed recommend the use of quinine in all cases of severe malaria. More recently the herb, *Artemisia annua* which has been in use for the treatment of malaria for some 2000 years, has been rediscovered as an effective drug for chloroquine-resistant malaria. The concentrated extract, qinghaosu, is in use in China.

Are there any precautions to be observed in the use of the non-prescription malaria chemoprophylactics?

As already discussed, use of the malaria chemoprophylactics including the non-prescription drugs during pregnancy is an area of concern. With chloroquine, recommended doses should not be exceeded as adverse reactions are then more likely. Renal and hepatic disease may lead to impaired clearance and hence increased toxicity with chloroquine. Caution is also required in the presence of porphyria, neurological and blood disorders, severe gastro-intestinal disease and in patients on anti-coagulant therapy. Transient visual effects may lead to problems when visual acuity is essential.

With pyrimethamine, recommended doses should also not be exceeded. Doses in excess of 25mg each week may lead to megaloblastic anaemia in patients also receiving co-trimoxazole. Co-administration of pyrimethamine and lorazepam may lead to hepatotoxicity. Because of pyrimethamine's mode of action, folate deficiency must be guarded against during pyrimethamine treatment.

Prominent adverse effects of the antimalarial agents are shown in Table 19.

Precautions and when to refer

(R) Pregnancy.

(R) Table 19.

(!) Porphyria, neurological and blood disorders, renal and hepatic disease, anticoagulant therapy and epilepsy with chloroquine.

(!) OTC antimalarials should be used only as prophylactics.

Products worth considering

Avloclor Tablets
(chloroquine)
Maloprim Tablets
(pyrimethamine,
dapsone)

Nivaquine Tablets
(chloroquine)
Nivaquine Syrup
(chloroquine)

Paludrine Tablets
(proguanil)
Primaquine Tablets
(primaquine)

The latest advice about drugs to be used in particular countries can be obtained from the malaria reference laboratory 0171-636-8636 or on 0171-388-9600 for prerecorded advice.

Mastitis

What is mastitis?

Sore nipples usually accompany breast feeding. In most common cases, the pain is a transient response to prolonged sucking of the nipples by the infant and resolves spontaneously. An emollient is usually all that is necessary. In some cases, the pain is due to an infection of the underlying tissues or lactating cells and inflammation is obvious (mastitis) Antibiotic therapy is usually then necessary.

Should antiseptic products be recommended for sore nipples?

Sore and cracked nipples occur in a large proportion of breast feeding mothers. This often leads to discontinuation of breast feeding, either because the pain becomes unbearable or because mastitis and abscesses develop. Therefore it is important to identify methods for preventing nipple trauma and reducing the risk of invasion of the lactating ducts by pathogenic micro-organisms. While antiseptic formulations appear to be a logical choice, a variety of as yet unproven remedies have been reported. Among these are initial wetting with breast milk, application of food oils or emollient creams and drying with corn flour.

Whether antiseptic formulations are any better than those unvalidated methods has not been fully assessed. Short-term trials using antiseptic formulations such as alcohol-based chlorhexidine sprays have yielded positive results in reducing the frequency and severity of nipple trauma in breast-feeding but these studies have generally tended to be short-term studies and the long-term implications of the use of the antiseptic sprays are not yet fully defined. Studies to evaluate the long-term effects of the antiseptic products on the breast flora are required to define whether there is any shift in the nature of the microbial flora and whether the short-term beneficial effects reported are sustained.

Despite these remaining questions, for mothers showing a proneness to develop sore nipples followed by mastitis, an antiseptic formulation is justifiable, but advice on proper breast feeding techniques and general hygiene should also be given. For the majority of mothers with no previous history of sore nipples or mastitis, pro-phylactic use of antiseptic formulations is not justified.

Precautions and when to refer

(R) When inflammation is present.

(R) Severe pain.

(!) Avoid iodine-containing products.

(!) Avoid hexachlorophane-containing products.

(!) Severe hypersensitivity reactions may occur with all antiseptic agents including chlorhexidine.

Products options

Kamillosan Ointment (chamomile)   Massé Breast Cream (emollient base)

Migraine

What is migraine?

Migraine is a complex disease entity characterized by severe headache and two types have been suggested. The first is characterized by headache accompanied by visual and/or gastro-intestinal disturbances. Attacks usually last for hours but in between episodes there is total freedom from symptoms. The second type is characterized by pain behind one, usually the same, eye which becomes red and watery. Attacks tend to occur for shorter periods but repeat attacks tend to persist for many weeks.

Migraine is a multifactorial disease and as with any such disease, various theories have been put forward for explaining the condition. Some authors believe that it is a food allergy, others that it is a cerebral disorder, while still others are of the view that it is due to a hormonal imbalance. That specific foods, stress and menstrual disturbances may all trigger migraine attacks suggests that no single theory is likely to be adequate for defining migraine.

Which is the best analgesic for migraine?

The best treatment for migraine will vary from patient to patient. Aspirin, ibuprofen and paracetamol are all useful initial therapies. However, gastric stasis is a feature of migraine and a soluble product is theoretically preferable. Indeed metoclopramide which accelerates gastric emptying is promoted either alone or in combination products for speeding up the absorption of analgesic compounds in migraine. Aspirin or paracetamol combinations with caffeine, cyclizine or codeine may also be worth trying although good trials to validate their claimed improved performance over the single analgesic compounds are lacking.

More recently, sumatriptan has been introduced as a treatment for migraine. Its mode of action is thought to be as a $5HT_1$ agonist. While it appears to be effective for acute attacks, its value in recurrent attacks is less well validated. This also applies to the older agents ergotamine and dihydroergotamine. These ergot derivatives are also now thought to owe their antimigraine effect to their $5HT_1$ agonist activity.

Are feverfew products useful for migraine?

A recent randomized, double-blind, cross-over, placebo-controlled trial using encapsulated feverfew leaves showed that the product was effective in reducing the mean number and severity of attacks over an 8-month period. Vomiting and visual analogue scores were also improved although the duration of the individual attacks was unaltered. While further confirmation of the results is required to assess the product's effectiveness relative to the better established remedies, the available results suggest that feverfew may be worth a try when standard therapies fail. During short-term therapy, mouth ulcers have been implicated as adverse reactions. Whether long-term use is likely to lead to any more serious adverse effects is as yet unknown.

Precautions and when to refer

(R) Patients on the combined contraceptive pill.

(R) Patients with persistent migraine.

(R) Hypertensive patients.

(!) Children under 12.

(!) See under analgesics.

(!) General recommendation

Analgesics are best taken immediately symptoms appear or are felt to be imminent.
Antihistamine-containing combination analgesics may exert some additional placebo effect but no more than those containing codeine.

Selected product options

Any full strength aspirin, paracetamol or ibuprofen-containing analgesic.

Migrafen Tablets (ibuprofen)   Librofem Tablets (ibuprofen)

As second-line products, codeine-containing combination products may be worthwhile.
   Cyclizine and buclizine-containing products may be acceptable as second-line agents too.

Femigraine Tablets (aspirin + cyclizine)   Migraleve 2 (paracetamol + codeine)
Migraleve 1 (paracetamol + codeine +
   buclizine)

Little is known about the value of isometheptene in migraine. The drug is a sympathomimetic agent and is therefore associated with adverse effects and interactions characteristic with this class of drugs. It is contra-indicated in glaucoma, severe cardiac and renal disease, porphyria, pregnancy and breast-feeding. It should be used with caution in the presence of cardiovascular, renal and hepatic disease, diabetes mellitus and hyperthyroidism and may cause dizziness.

Midrid Capsules (paracetamol; isometheptene)

Mouth ulcers

What are mouth ulcers?

Mouth ulcers are one of the commonest oral lesions seen in general practice. Over a fifth of the general population are affected and women seem to be more susceptible than men. There seems to be a genetic influence on susceptibility to mouth ulcers but the exact mode of transmission is as yet unknown.

Are canker sores the same as mouth ulcers?

Canker sores is the North American terminology for mouth ulcers. Alternative terms commonly used to describe the same clinical problem are aphthous ulcers and recurrent aphthous stomatitis.

What causes mouth ulcers?

The aetiology of mouth ulcers is still unclear and both endogenous precipitating factors and micro-organisms have been postulated. In particular, a hypersensitivity to antigenic components of *Streptococcus sanguinis*, a pleomorphic alpha-haemolytic bacteria, has been suggested. Mouth ulcers are distinct from cold sores which are known to be caused by the herpes simplex virus. Precipitating factors suggested include physical irritation, emotional stress, irritant or allergenic foods, hormonal changes and vitamin deficiency but none are of proven significance.

Can drugs induce mouth-ulcers?

Yes, it would appear so. Patients receiving chemotherapy or radiation or both may develop mouth ulcers. It has been suggested that this problem may be caused by the non-specific action of the cytotoxic drugs on the rapidly dividing cells of the basal epithelium. The mucosal ulcerations are usually preceded by dryness of the mouth, burning and tingling of the lips and generalized pain in the mucosal membranes. The term mucositis is often applied to this syndrome. Methyldopa has also been claimed to induce mouth ulcers. A list of drugs associated with mouth ulcers and other buccal adverse reactions is given in Table 20.

How can cold sores be distinguished from mouth ulcers?

A recurring lesion at the mucocutaneous junction of the lips and adjacent skin strongly suggests a cold sore (see section on cold sores). Mouth ulcers are restricted to the buccal cavity. Differential diagnosis becomes difficult when the lesions are in

Table 20 Drugs which may cause adverse reactions in the buccal cavity.

Aphthous ulcers:

Allopurinol	Hydroxychloroquine	Penicillamine
Dapsone	Isoniazid	Penicillin
Frusemide	Methyldopa	Propranolol
Gold	Naproxen	Streptomycin
Griseofulvin	Phenothiazines	Tetracycline
Hydralazine	Phenothiazines	Thiazides

Dry mouth

Amiloride	Emepronium bromide	Nortriptyline
Amitriptyline	Etretinate	Orphenadrine
Atropine	Flavoxate	Oxypertine
Azatadine	Fluphenazine	Pargyline
Benzhexol	Fluspirilene	Pericyazine
Benztropine	Hydroxyzine	Phenazocine
Biperiden	Hyoscine butylbromide	Phenelzine
Bromocriptine	Imipramine	Phenindamine
Busulphan	Indoramin	Phenylbutazone
Carbamazepine	Ipratropium	Pirenzepine
Chlormezanone	Iproniazid	Poldine
Chlorpromazine	Isocarboxazid	Potassium clorazepate
Clemastine	Isotretinoin	Prazosin
Clobazam	Ketamine	Prochlorperazine
Clomipramine	Ketotifen	Procyclidine
Clonazepam	Levodopa	Promazine
Clonidine	Lofepramine	Propantheline
Cyclizine	Maprotiline	Pyridostigmine
Cyproheptadine	Mazindol	Sulphasalazine
Desipramine	Mepyramine	Suxamethonium
Dexamphetamine	Methixene	Thioridazine
Dicyclomine	Methotrimeprazine	Tranycypromine
Diethylpropion	Methyldopa	Trazodone
Diphenylpyraline	Nabilone	Triamterene
Disopyramide	Nadolol	Trifluoperazine
Dothiepin	Nalbuphine	Trimeprazine
Doxapram	Nefopam	Trimipramine
Doxepin	Neostigmine	Viloxazine
Edrephonium	Nomifensine	

Dysphagia (difficulty in swallowing):
Atropine
Doxycycline
Vindesine

(See also oesophagitis)

Gingival hypertrophy:
Cyclosporin
Phenytoin

Table 20 Drugs which may cause adverse reactions in the buccal cavity (*continued*).

Halitosis:

Dimethyl	Any drug inhibiting
Sulphoxide	salivary excretion
Garlic extracts	(see dry mouth)

Inflammation: (*See* stomatitis)

Mouth ulcers: (*See* aphthous ulcers)

Oesophagitis:

Co-trimoxazole	Fludrocortisone
Dactinomycin	Hydrocortisone
Dexamethasone	Indomethacin
Doxycycline	Prednisolone
Emepronium bromide	Triamcinolone

(*See also* dysphagia)

Salivary gland disorders: (*See* dry mouth)

Stomatitis (inflammation of oral mucosa):

Allopurinol	Diflunisal	Mercaptopurine
Amitriptyline	Emepronium bromide	Methotrexate
Amasacrine	Epirubicin	Mithramycin
Bleomycin	Fenoprofen	Penicillamine
Captopril	Flurbiprofen	Sulindac
Chlorambucil	Hydroxyurea	Sulphasalazine
Chloramphenicol	Ifosfamide	Treosulphan
Cyclophosphamide	Indomethacin	Vinglastine
Cytarabine	Lomustine	Vincristine
Dactinomycin	Melphalan	Vindesine

Stains: (*See* teeth stains)

Taste disturbance:

Allopurinol	Flurazepam
Amiodarone	Levodopa
Amitriptyline	Metronidazole
Calcitonin	Nortriptyline
Captopril	Penicillamine
Ceftazidime	Procainamide
Cisplatin	Propantheline
Doxepin	Tinidazole
Enalapril	Triazolam

Teeth stains:

Chlorhexidine	Erythromycin
Chlortetracycline	Oxytetracycline
Clomocycline	Stannous fluoride

Table 20   Drugs which may cause adverse reactions in the buccal cavity (*continued*).

Demeclocycline	Tetracycline
Doxycycline	
(*See also* stains)	
Thirst:	
Acetazolamide	Dicyclomine
Atropine	Lithium
(*See also* dry mouth)	

the mouth. With cold sores the lesions are papular and vesicular, while in mouth ulcers the lesions are slightly depressed and are surrounded by an intense erythematous halo. Both conditions are intensely painful and are associated with bad breath.

What is the natural history of mouth ulcers?

One striking feature of mouth ulcers is their sudden appearance. Intense pain is usually the first feature noted by the mouth ulcer patient. The lesions normally enlarge to about 5 mm but in severe cases may grow to as much as 30 mm in diameter. The pain is severe enough to interfere with eating and speaking. Resolution of the ulcers is usually as abrupt as their onset, within 7–14 days after their first appearance. The ulcers usually occur singly. Lesions which persist beyond 3 weeks should be investigated.

How should mouth ulcers be managed?

As the exact cause is unknown, only symptomatic treatment is available. Warm saline mouthwashes are cheap and readily prepared at home. An antiseptic mouthwash may also help, particularly if halitosis is a problem, but the most effective product is likely to be an anaesthetic gel. Hydrocortisone pellets are often prescribed as are mucoadhesive bases (Orabase). Zinc sulphate, lactobacilli, contraceptive pills, carbenoxolone, sucralfate and sodium cromoglycate are all insufficiently validated therapies for mouth ulcers to justify recommendation.

Precautions and when to refer

Mouth ulcers persisting for longer than 3 weeks (to exclude other pathology including malignancy, blood dyscrasia and erythema multiforme).

Non-painful lesions (including any lump, thickening or red or white patches (to exclude possible malignancy).

(R) Difficulty in chewing or swallowing not associated with a sore lesion.

(R) Any sore that bleeds easily.

(!) General recommendations

Local anaesthetics will provide short-term relief.
Topical corticosteroids will reduce inflammation.
Antiseptics are not useful in mouth-ulcers.
Carbenoxolone is a second-line agent.

Selected product options

Adcortyl in Orabase	Calgel	Ulc-Aid
Anbesol gel	Dentinox gel	

Nappy rash

What is nappy rash?

Nappy rash is characterized by skin maceration, erythema and scaling in the nappy area. It is often referred to as diaper rash. The rash is generally thought to be a dermatitis induced by irritants present in urine or faeces. The most widely held theory is that micro-organisms within the nappy area produce enzymes which split urinary urea into irritant ammonia. For this reason, nappy rash is often called ammoniacal dermatitis. Recent studies, however, suggest that ammonia is unlikely to be the prime irritant but that the alkaline pH it produces activates faecal proteases and lipases. The skin is thereby damaged and its permeability to irritants is increased. The yet to be identified irritants then cause the classical symptoms of dermatitis.

Which micro-organisms are involved in nappy rash?

The urea-splitting organism is known as *Brevibacterium ammoniagenes*. Recent studies have shown that by 72 hours most nappy rashes show positive cultures to *Candida albicans*. *Staphylococcus aureus* is also more commonly isolated from the nappy area in the presence of nappy rash than in its absence.

How should nappy rash be managed?

The acute attack is best treated by proper cleansing of the nappy area and air exposure of the affected area, to reduce maceration of the skin. A water-repellent cream, white soft paraffin or Zinc Oxide and Castor Oil Ointment can then be applied to the dry area before the wearing of the next nappy. This should be repeated after each subsequent nappy change. In the presence of skin lesions, anti-bacterial and anti-candidal cover is useful and an imidazole anti-candidal (miconazole, clotrimazole, econazole) cream would be an ideal choice. Antiseptic creams containing chlorhexidine or quaternary ammonium salts may be helpful but have generally been inadequately evaluated in nappy rash. After resolution of the lesions, prophylactic use of a water-repellent formulation such as white soft paraffin or a silicone cream is recommended.

Is hydrocortisone cream useful in nappy rash?

Hydrocortisone cream is helpful in reducing the inflammation which may be seen in the more severe cases of nappy rash. However, treatment should be limited to no more than 1 week. Note that nappy rash is not a licensed indication for non-prescription hydrocortisone creams.

Are boric acid and hydrargraphen formulations still justifiable for nappy rash?

Both active ingredients are toxic when absorbed and neither has been shown to be more effective than the safer alternatives already discussed. Continued use of boric acid and hydrargraphen in nappy rash is therefore no longer justified.

Some health visitors recommend the application of fresh egg white to nappy lesions. Is this beneficial?

Egg readily causes sensitization when injected into the systemic circulation. Its use on raw lesions is to be strongly discouraged.

Are antihistamines useful in nappy rash?

Topical antihistamines may sensitize and should therefore be avoided, particularly when the skin barrier is impaired. Their use in nappy rash is therefore not rational.

Are dusting powders useful in drying out the nappy area?

Talc and dusting powders are widely used by mothers. Some authors have expressed concern about entrapment of potentially toxic particulate matter in exposed areas but the risk seems to be minimal. On the other hand, there is little justification in promoting the use of the powders in nappy rash.

Is it true that breast feeding may protect babies against nappy rash?

Surveys have in fact shown this to be the case. The proposed reason is that breast fed infants produce a lower and less irritant urine output than bottle fed infants. A higher urinary pH is thought to activate faecal proteases and lipases, which are damaging to the skin. Irritants can therefore, as a result, inflict more damage to the underlying tissues.

Precautions and when to refer

 When rash not confined to nappy area.

 When secondary infection present and rash is severe.

Product options

Compendial products

Aqueous Cream	Zinc and Castor Oll Ointment	Zinc and Castor Oil Cream

Proprietary products
Conotrane Cream (benzalkonium chloride, dimethicone)
Drapolene Cream (benzalkonium chloride, cetrimide)
Kamillosan Ointment (chamomile extracts)
Metanium Ointment (titanium dioxide, peroxide, salicylate and tannate in silicone basis)
Sudocrem (benzyl alcohol, benzyl benzoate, benzyl cinnamate)
Vasogen Cream (dimethiscone, calamine, zinc oxide)

Ovulation tests

How do ovulation tests work?

The recently introduced OTC ovulation tests (e.g. First Response) work by monitoring the level of luteinising hormone (LH) in urine. Unlike gonadotrophin, the marker used in pregnancy tests, luteinising hormone is present in the urine throughout the menstrual cycle irrespective of whether the woman is pregnant or not. However, ovulation is preceded by a significant surge in urinary levels of LH (Figure 10) and it is this surge which provides the basis for the ovulation tests. The luteinising hormone is assayed by an immunoassay similar to the pregnancy tests, and to enable ready visualization of results the final step is usually an enzyme-linked colour reaction which must be matched, at a fixed time, against standard colour charts.

When should the ovulation tests be performed?

The tests are usually performed from about 3 days ahead of the predicted ovulation time, based on the previous lengths of the menstrual cycle. Thus, a women with the standard 28 day cycle would start testing from day 12 of her cycle. Many women of low fertility would have irregular periods and for these women, the shortest cycle is usually recommended for use in predicting the best timing for the tests.

Can ovulation tests be used for contraception?

Theoretically ovulation tests should provide elegant non-invasive methods for contraception. However, sperm can survive for up to 72 hours in the vagina and currently available methods can predict ovulation only 36 hours ahead of time. Therefore, the tests would be highly unreliable for contraception.

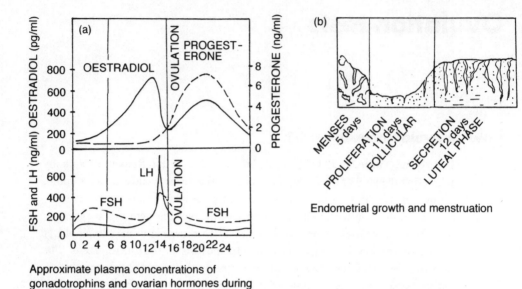

Approximate plasma concentrations of gonadotrophins and ovarian hormones during the normal female cycle

Endometrial growth and menstruation

Fig. 10   Hormonal and endometrial changes throughout the menstrual cycle.

Product options

Clearplan One Step Ovulation Test

Pregnancy tests

How do pregnancy tests work?

Following implantation of the ovum, the syncytial trophoblast cells secrete human chorionic gonadotrophin (HCG). This hormone ensures that the corpus luteum does not involute as is normal at the end of each cycle, in the absence of pregnancy. HCG is therefore a very specific marker of pregnancy and all commonly used pregnancy tests rely on its detection. A number of specific methods are used for detecting HCG, including the following.

(1) *The slide tests.* In these tests, a suspension of latex coated with HCG is supplied together with a solution of HCG antibody. In the absence of urinary HCG, the latex particles react with the HCG antibody to produce agglutination or clumping on the slide. In the presence of urinary HCG the antibodies react with it instead of with the HCG-coated latex particles and a creamy non-agglutinated mixture is seen on the slide.

(2) *The tube tests.* In these tests, a suspension of red blood cells coated with HCG is supplied together with a solution of HCG antibody. In the presence of urinary HCG, the antibody reacts with it to leave the HCG-coated red blood cells to settle as a ring at the bottom of the test tube. In the absence of pregnancy and hence of HCG, agglutination between the HCG-coated red blood cells and the HCG antibody takes place and the distinct ring is absent.

(3) *Radio immunoassays (RIA).* These are highly sensitive and because measurements of radioactivity are involved, tests are confined to specialist laboratories. The tests are essentially based on interaction of HCG with radioactive anti-HCG tracers.

(4) *Enzyme immunoassays.* These have sensitivities similar to those of radio immunoassays but have the advantage of being suitable for use by untrained persons. Instead of a radioactive tracer, an enzyme is used to interact with HCG. The enzyme complex is then used to produce a colour change indicative of pregnancy. The most up to date pregnancy tests are based on such enzyme immunoassays. Typically, a sampler to which HCG antibody has been immolised is placed in a urine sample. If the urine contains HCG, then the latter is taken up by the sampler. Excess urine is washed off and the sampler to which HCG is sorbed, is then dipped into a well containing anti-HCG antibody linked to an enzyme such as alkaline phosphatase. The enzyme now attached to the sampler is then used to develop a colour in a third well. A colour therefore indicates a positive result.

How accurate are the modern pregnancy tests?

The manufacturers claim 99% accuracy for their tests. Although the accuracy achievable in actual use is likely to be lower than this figure due to non-adherence to manufactures' instructions, there is no reason to suspect that the accuracy is substantially less than the manufacturers' claims.

What are monoclonal antibodies?

Monoclonal antibodies are antibodies which are specific against a single antigenic locus on the HCG molecule. To understand how this is done consider an animal which is innoculated with HCG. Each lymphocyte responds to produce antibodies against one single antigenic determinant. If the HCG molecules has n antigenic determinants then n different types of antibodies will be formed. Some of the HCG antigenic determinants are the same as those found in other molecules, notably luteinising hormone. Therefore, if antibodies raised against HCG in this way were used, the mixture will show poor specificity.

Any primed lymphocyte will subdivide to produce identical cells (clones) all producing identical antibodies. By identifying lymphocytes which produce a specific antibody, and isolating them, pure or monoclonal antibodies can be produced. The breakthrough in mass producing monoclonal antibodies came when Kohler and Milstein developed cell-fusion techniques for doing so. Essentially, their technique involved fusing primed lymphocytes with myeloma cells which can be cultured and divided rapidly *in vitro*. Some of the hybrid cells (hybridomas) retain the ability to produce only one type of antibody. Therefore selective growth of these hybridomas and harvesting of the single determinant antibodies increases the specificity of the anti-HCG antibodies. Specificity by itself is however not sufficient. The affinity of the antibody for HCG must be sufficiently high to ensure that the antiserum has adequate sensitivity.

Do monoclonal antibodies improve the performance of pregnancy tests?

Polyclonal antibodies tend to be non-specific and may react with a number of components, other than HCG, found in urine. By using monoclonal antibodies, specificity and reactivity can be improved. The latest pregnancy tests, for example, use antibodies directed specifically against antigenic determinants on the β subunit of HCG. Coupling of such an antigenic locus with a second elsewhere on the HCG may lead to highly specific bridging and precipation of the complexes formed.

Why should an early morning urine sample preferably be used in pregnancy testing?

Early morning urine samples tend to have higher levels of HCG because of the usual absence of voiding of the bladder during the night. Therefore, the chances of detecting low levels of HCG early in pregnancy are improved by using an early morning urine sample.

How soon can a pregnancy be detected?

With the most up to date tests (e.g. Clearblue and Discover Colour) pregnancy can be detected virtually on the day of the missed period. All the other current tests should identify a pregnancy within a week of the missed period. Therefore, in practice, pregnancies can be identified by all the tests as soon as the women normally want them to be.

Precautions and when to refer

 Refer patients with a positive test.

 Patients who repeatedly seek pregnancy tests.

Product options

Clearblue Home Pregnancy Test Kit
Confirm Home Pregnancy Test Kit
Discover 2 Pregnancy Test Kit
Discover Today

Evatest Pregnancy Test Kit
Predictor Colour Pregnancy Test Kit
Predictor Pregnancy Test Kit

Premenstrual tension

What is premenstrual tension?

Premenstrual tension (PMT) or premenstrual syndrome (PMS) refers to a group of symptoms which many women suffer from during the premenstrual period. Those symptoms include irritability, fluid retention, unusual cravings, disturbed sleep, anxiety and headache. There is as yet no generally accepted aetiology for the syndrome. Theories put forward include imbalance in oestrogen–progesterone activity, deficiency in essential fatty-acids, and excessive secretions of neuropeptides and prostaglandins.

What OTC treatments are available for PMT?

Given that there are a number of theories put forward to account for PMT, it is not surprising that the treatments proposed are also numerous. These include steroidal anti-inflammatory analgesics to inhibit prostaglandin formation, pyridoxine to improve mood disturbance, evening primrose oil to correct fatty-acid deficiency, and ammonium chloride to reduce fluid retention. None of these is consistently effective. Excessive doses may cause toxicity; pyridoxine leading to neurosensory problems and ammonium chloride to gastric irritation and electrolyte imbalance.

Precautions and when to refer_____

(R) Presence of very severe symptoms.

(R) Severe menstrual problems.

(!) Excessive pyridoxine intake leads to neurotoxic symptoms.

Product options _____

Aquaban Tablets (caffeine, ammonium chloride)
Efamol High Strength Premenstrual Pack (Evening Primrose Oil, Vitamins C, B$_6$ and E, biotin, zinc, magnesium, niacin)

Pressure sores

What are pressure sores?

As their name suggests, pressure sores are lesions arising from application of prolonged pressure to specific areas of the body. The sores are usually associated with prolonged bed rest and areas commonly affected are the buttocks and the heels.

Are pressure sores the same as bed sores?

Both terms are indeed synonymous and the terms decubitus ulcers and leg ulcers have also been used for the condition.

What factors other than pressure increase the likelihood of pressure sores?

Friction and moisture are commonly regarded as contributing factors to the development of pressure sores as is the increased fibrinolytic activity observed in a variety of diseases. Infections organisms may also be ulcerogenic and may certainly cause spread of the initial pressure-induced lesion. Indeed putrefactive activity is commonly encountered with pressure sores.

What is the pathophysiology of the condition?

Pressure leads to the underlying tissues being deprived of oxygen. Inflammatory reactions lead to oedema and subsequently to necrosis of the affected tissues. Secondary bacterial infection and continued pressure eventually lead to an open ulcer.

Are some pressure sores easier to manage than others?

Recovery from pressure sores depends on the extent of the lesions and the state of general health of the patient. The severity of pressure sores is commonly classified under four grades. At stage one, the lesion is no more than an erythematous area which still blanches on application of light pressure. At stage two this blanching response is absent and inflammation of the underlying issues is obvious; pain intensifies. At stage three, erosion of the epidermis is obvious and may be encrusted. Further spread of the lesion into the deeper tissues leads to exposure of the dermis, and even the muscles and bone may be visible. At this grade four stage, healing is obviously most difficult. If the patient is debilitated or diabetic, recovery is even more prolonged because of impaired regenerative capacity. The incontinent patient presents particularly difficult problems because of contact dermatitis (see nappy rash) and secondary bacterial contamination. For these difficult or high risk patients prevention is particularly important.

How are pressure sores prevented?

Frequent positional changes are an obvious approach. At least half-hourly changes in position are recommended but sadly for most patients this is a difficult goal to achieve without specialized mechanical devices. Water mattresses, sheepskin pads and polyurethane foam paddings have been used with some limited success. General hygiene of the affected area and prevention of incontinence help. Good skin care is essential.

How should an established ulcer be managed?

Relief of pressure is clearly essential as is regular cleaning to remove tissue debris and necrotic tissues. A wide array of products is available but the first logical approach is the use of plenty of water. An isotonic salt solution may reduce stinging. A final rinse with an antibacterial product such as chlorhexidine solution or a solution of a quaternary ammonium disinfectant (cetrimide, benzalkonium) may reduce the likelihood of secondary infections. Povidone-iodine and mercurials should not be used because of potential systemic toxicity. Hypochlorite solutions (Eusol) are still widely used and plain Eusol solution is preferable to the commonly prescribed Eusol and liquid paraffin as fatty bases may retard wound healing. Occlusive dressings should be avoided to prevent further maceration. Hydrocolloid adhesive dressings and gas permeable polyurethane film dressings have however been shown to be beneficial.

Are peroxide and permanganate solutions still recommended?

Both are still regularly prescribed and are probably as useful as any other cleansing solution although there is some concern about the cytotoxicity of oxidizing agents in general. The release of oxygen by hydrogen peroxide when in contact with tissue exudates may help to loosen debris.

Do ascorbic acid and zinc sulphate supplements help?

Both agents are known to participate in wound healing. In the presence of deficiency, supplements are helpful but generally there is little evidence that either agent promotes healing. Low dose supplements of ascorbic acid are safe and there is little need to strongly discourage their use.

Do sugar granules and gelatin promote epithelialization?

Concentrated sugar solutions may exert an antibacterial activity through an osmotic effect or so called alteration in water activity but there is little evidence that either sugar or gelatin are helpful adjuncts to promote epithelialization in pressure sores.

Precautions and when to refer

(R) Worsening pressure sores.

(R) Evidence of secondary infection.

(R) Diabetic patients.

(R) Any patient not also under constant care.

(!) What general advice should one give?

Sufferers should be repositioned or reposition themselves as frequently as possible.
The head of the bed should not be elevated.
Pressure on bony prominences should be minimized with pillows or foam cushions.
The skin should be inspected regularly.
When bathing, hot water should be avoided and only mild cleansing agents used.
Maceration of the skin due to soiling or incontinence should be minimized by rapid cleansing.

Product options

Compendial products
Zinc and Castor Oil Cream

Proprietary products
Conotrane Cream (benzalkonium chloride, dimethicone)
Drapolene Cream (benzalkonium chloride)
Morhulin Ointment (zinc oxide, cod liver oil)

Sprilon Spray (dimethicone, zinc oxide)
Vasogen Cream (zinc oxide, calamine, dimethicone)

Psoriasis

What is psoriasis and how should it be managed?

Psoriasis is characterized by skin thickening and scaling. The lesions are sharply demarcated and usually present with silvery scales superimposed on salmon-pink plaques (thick patches). The lesions tend to be more persistent than eczema. The aetiology is poorly understood and there is a strong hereditary component. Treatment of psoriasis is difficult. Mild conditions respond to emollients. Persistent cases may benefit from salicylic acid, coal tar or dithranol-based products. More latterly, vitamin D_3 analogues such as calcipotriol and tracalcitol are being regarded as first line agents in those not responsive to simple emollients and tar products.

Precautions and when to refer

 Psoriasis is difficult to treat. Except for the mildest cases, the patient should be referred.

 Avoid use of topical hydrocortisone.

Product options

First line agents: Emollients, Coal tar products

Alphosyl Cream	Cocois Scalp Ointment	Pragmatar Cream
Alphosyl 2 in 1 Shampoo	Gelcosal Gel	Psoriderm Cream
Carbo-Dome Cream	Gelcotar Gel	PsoriGel
Clinitar Cream		

Bath preparations containing coal tar

Coal tar solution	Pixol bath oil	Psoriderm bath emulsion
Basneum with tar oil	Polytar emollient bath additive	

Second-line agents: Dithranol-containing products

Dithranol Paste (plus salicylic acid)	Psorin Scalp Gel (plus salicylic acid and methyl salicylate)
Dithrocream	
Psorin Ointment (plus coal tar)	Psorin Ointment (plus salicylic acid and coal tar)

Scabies

What is scabies?

Scabies is an infestation by the mite *Sarcoptes scabiei*. The mite, which is not readily seen with the naked eye, usually burrows into the skin, typically on the hands, the wrists, the elbows, the penis and scrotum. The mite causes intense itchiness which is characteristic of the disease. Secondary bacterial infections may lead to pustules, impetigo and crusting. Crusted scabies, which is often seen among the elderly and the immunocompromised, is often mistaken for eczema and may act as a source of infestation.

How is scabies spread?

Close contact with an infected person is usually required as the mite dies within 2 days of leaving the host. Theoretically, cross-infestation may take place through bedding, towels and underclothing but this is usually accepted as being rare except within the confines of a family, nursing home or other closed institution. Transmission to sexual partners occurs readily.

How should scabies be treated?

Application of a suitable scabicide to the whole body but omitting the head is required. An antipruritic or oral antihistamine may help relieve itching in the early stages of treatment. Family members or sexual partners should normally also be treated simultaneously. Crotamiton, gamma benzene hexachloride and monosulfiram are the only preparations used for the treatment of scabies. Gamma benzene hexachloride is generally regarded as being the more effective compound although systemic toxicity has followed its use. Crotamiton is less effective but has useful antipruritic properties. Monosulfiram, now relatively rarely used, may behave like disulfiram in its interaction with alcohol.

Precautions and when to refer

(*See under* lice.)

Product options

First-line agents
Derbac M (malathion)   Suleo-M Lotion (malathion)
Prioderm M (malathion)   Lyclear Dermal Cream (permethrin)
Quellada M liquid (malathion)

Second-line agents
Ascabiol Emulsion (benzyl benzoate)   Benzyl benzoate Application BP

Shingles

Shingles is still an enigmatic condition and treatment and prevention still inadequate. Relative to other viral infections such as the common cold and warts, shingles is a rare condition. Yet every pharmacist with some experience of general practice has no doubt met a number of patients with shingles who have sought help and advice on its management.

What is shingles?

Shingles is caused by the *varicella-zoster* (VZ) virus which also causes chickenpox. The generally accepted theory is that following an attack of chickenpox, some of the viral particles remain viable but dormant. Years later, trigger factors reactivate them.

What activates the latent virus?

Local trauma is clearly one cause. More generally it is probable that the viruses become active because defence mechanisms which previously controlled the virus weaken and fail. Patients on cancer chemotherapy are often vulnerable because of the exogenously induced depression of the immune response. Corticosteroids may also activate shingles by the same mechanism. More recently, it has been suggested that antihistamines may also be responsible for activating the disease but the data are much too isolated to draw any conclusion at this stage.

How contagious is shingles?

Little is known about the mode of transmission of the virus but observed clustering of cases in some instances suggests that perhaps the disease may be infectious but of low infectivity.

How can one tell that one is suffering from shingles?

The most characteristic feature of shingles is the lesions which usually appear on the chest or face. Severe pain is virtually always present in adult patients at all stages of the disease and occurs several days before lesions are seen. The lesions bleed readily and become highly encrusted. Secondary infections may set in.

How long will the condition last?

Typically, the adult patient can expect to be in discomfort for weeks rather than days. Pain may persist for months. In children, the condition resolves much more readily and is usually mild.

Can one catch shingles from patients with chickenpox?

This is not likely although the reverse, that is catching chickenpox from patients with shingles, is a real possibility. Shingles is a reactivated infection while chickenpox is usually a first infection.

Is it true that the disease only occurs in the elderly?

While it is true that the elderly are particularly prone to the disease because of a weakening of the immune response associated with the ageing process, shingles can affect individuals of all ages.

Is it possible for patients to suffer from shingles on more than one occasion?

Yes but this is generally rare. An incidence of 1–2% of reinfection has been reported.

How severe are possible complications?

Severe complications are relatively rare although long-term pain is common. The affected site may also become anaesthetized.

Each year a number of deaths are recorded from *varicella* infections. Most of these are, however, probably in immunocompromised hosts. The major complications of the disease are pneumonia and encephalitis. When the facial nerve is involved, vision can be affected and Bell's palsy, a condition characterized by loss of control of the facial muscles, is also a possibility.

Reye's syndrome, a condition characterized by sudden central nervous system symptoms, liver degeneration and a high mortality rate, is known to be associated with recent viral infections, particularly influenza and VZ infections. The latter is, of course, highly pertinent in the present context. The controversial suggestion has also been made that in the presence of these viral infections, salicylates ingestion may lead to the syndrome. The controversy has not yet been resolved, but since satisfactory alternative weak analgesics are so easily available, it is clearly not prudent to use aspirin in such patients on current evidence.

How effective are current treatments?

Idoxuridine in dimethylsulphoxide is perhaps the most effective therapy currently available, although even with this drug success can be unpredictable. Treatment is best started early in order to minimize the chances of complications. Acyclovir is showing high promise when used parenterally for the treatment of patients at high risk of developing severe complications and when recurrence may be a problem. The topical formulation used in general practice medicine is aimed at patients with herpes simplex rather than at patients with VZ infections.

Is there any link between herpes simplex and the varicella-zoster virus?

On culture, the two types of viruses can easily be shown to be different. Yet, ultrastructurally, they are similar and induce the same histopathological responses. The lesions are often similar although herpes simplex tends to affect areas covered with mucous membranes such as the lips and genitals. The two viruses may occur concurrently in the same lesions. Genital herpes may be as unpleasant as shingles.

Can one be vaccinated against shingles?

In the otherwise healthy person, shingles does not normally present a major threat and because of this, the search for effective vaccines has not been very intense. More recently, however, recognition of the danger which the disease represents to the immunosuppressed patient has led to increased activity in this field. Success, however, is still elusive. Clearly such a vaccine will probably only be useful in a small group of potential patients. Its wider use to prevent chickenpox may lead to problems of postponing the disease to adulthood when the risk of severe complications is higher.

Is there any non-prescription medication for the long-suffering patient who has lost all faith in prescribed medication?

Effective doses of analgesics are required. Normally stronger analgesics than are available over the counter will be needed. Paracetamol either alone or in combination with codeine may be worth a try although the evidence for any synergistic activity with the combination product is limited.

What is post-herpetic neuralgia and what causes it?

One of the most unpleasant features of herpes zoster is the pain which almost invariably follows the healing of the herpetic lesions. This painful condition is referred to as post-herpetic neuralgia. The pathogenesis is still unknown but an excess of unopposed unmyelinated fibre activity due to a reduction in the number of large myelinated axons has been suggested. A recent alternative theory is that the virus infection causes abnormal impulses to be fired from the dorsal root ganglion neurons.

Precautions and when to refer

 Early referral of patients with shingles is strongly advised.

 Ensure that additional analgesics are not given if patient is already under prescribed analgesics.

Product options

Axsain Cream (capsaicin)
(See analgesics (oral).)

Sleep aids

Are non-prescription sleep-aids justified?

This is an extremely difficult question to answer. In principle, it can be argued that self-limiting insomnia should be managed conservatively without the use of any hypnotic agent. In practice, however, many individuals are helped by a short course of sleep-inducing medication and these individuals would insist that their health status is much improved as a result of such therapy. The problem is even more complex when the question is whether such therapy should be self-prescribed. Regulatory authorities are, however, sufficiently convinced to grant product licences to a number of manufacturers for sleep-aid products. The rational approach appears to be to manage insomnia non-pharmacologically first, perhaps by counting sheep or soldiers. If this fails, placebo therapy with an appropriate herbal tea may work; if not, a non-prescription antihistamine may be recommended. If no success follows then prescribed medication seems appropriate.

Is promethazine effective as a sleep aid?

Promethazine, in common with many H_1 antihistamine compounds, exerts a central nervous system depressant activity, including the well-known drowsiness. Therefore in principle promethazine should help induce sleep. Indeed promethazine has been included in teething remedies for a long time with the objective of inducing sleep. Some clinical trials show that the drug is better than a placebo as a sleep aid and does not interfere with the quality of sleep. However, tolerance may develop with long-term use.

Is promethazine safe?

Promethazine appears to be a relatively safe phenothiazine. Anticholinergic effects may however be pronounced and the occasional photosensitivity reactions have been reported. The drug is transferred across the placenta but no teratogenic effects have been reported. However, as a general safety measure, all drugs should be avoided during pregnancy if at all possible. In overdose, disorientation and agitation have been reported.

Is valerian useful as a sleep-aid?

Insomnia is subject to a high placebo effect and there is little doubt that at least some people will be helped by the herb. However, there is also some evidence indicating that the product may be more effective than a placebo although confirmatory evidence is still necessary.

Is tryptophan useful as a sleep aid?

There is some evidence that tryptophan may be effective as a sleep aid although clinical trials have yielded contradictory results. However recently, tryptophan has been associated with an epidemic of eosinophiliamyalgia syndrome, a potentially fatal condition. For this reason it has been withdrawn from OTC use in the United Kingdom.

Is melatonin a useful hypnotic?

There is evidence that melatonin participates in the maintenance of circadian rhythms including sleep regulation. Elderly insomniacs have significantly lower serum melatonin concentrations than normal controls and ingestion of melatonin appears to increase the speed of falling asleep and the duration and quality of sleep. More clinical trials are required to define its precise value as a hypnotic but the early results are encouraging. Melatonin is not currently available as a health supplement or licensed product in the UK.

Is diphenhydramine a useful hypnotic?

In common with promethazine, diphenhydramine (another H_1 antihistamine) induces drowsiness, and may therefore be useful as a mild hypnotic.

Product options

Antihistamine-containing products
Medinex Syrup (diphenhydramine)
Nytol Tablets (diphenhydramine)
Nytol One-a-Night Tablets
  (diphenhydramine)
Phenergan Nightime Tablets
  (promethazine)
Sominex Tablets (promethazine)

Herbal remedies
Kalms Tablets (humulus lupulus, gentiana lutea, valeriana officinalis)
Natrasleep Tablets (humulus lupulus, valeriana officinalis)
Potter's Nodoff Passiflora Tablets (passiflora)

Sore throats

What causes sore throats?

Most sore throats are caused by infection of the tonsils, larynx or pharynx and the resulting inflammation (tonsillitis, laryngitis and pharyngitis) of those tissues.

Viruses are most commonly involved and there is no reliable visual marker for separating viral sore throats from those of bacterial origin. The more frequent bacteria involved are the beta-haemolytic streptococci, *Streptococcus pneumoniae* and *Haemophilus influenzae*. When such streptococci are involved, there is a risk of systemic invasion leading to acute rheumatic fever and glomerulonephritis. Sore throat is also a non-specific symptom of malignancy and of course over-use of the vocal chords.

How should sore throats be managed?

Acute sore throats accompanying upper respiratory tract infection by the common cold viruses usually resolve spontaneously within 3 days. Symptomatic relief with anaesthetic lozenges and sprays is therefore helpful. Oral analgesics will also help. Oral gargles may help to freshen the mouth. Antibacterial products are unlikely to alter the course of sore throats. It is important to refer cases of sore throat with unusual presentation (see below).

Precautions and when to refer

(R) Sore throats in children, particularly if severe.

(R) Sore throats accompanied by a high temperature as this may indicate a streptococcal infection which will need antibiotic cover.

(R) Persistent sore throats (> 5 days) as this may be indicative of other disease.

(R) Severe sore throats, particularly if of sudden onset as there is an increased likelihood of a bacterial infection.

(!) Avoid over-use of phenol-containing gargles as severe adverse effects have been reported.

Product options

Anaesthetic and anaesthetic-antibacterial products
AAA mouth and throat spray (benzocaine)
Bradosol Plus Lozenges (lignocaine, domiphen bromide)
DeWitt's Throat Lozenges (benzocaine, cetylpyridinium chloride)
Dequacaine Lozenges (benzocaine, dequalinium chloride)
Eludril Spray (amethocaine, chlorhexidine gluconate)
Strepsils Dual Action Lozenges (lignocaine, amylmetacresol, dichlorobenzyl alcohol)
Tyrozets Lozenges (benzocaine tyrothricin)
Vicks Ultra Chloraseptic Spray (benzocaine)

Antibacterial products
Betadine Gargle (povidone-iodine)
Bradosol Lozenges (benzalkonium chloride)
Dequadin Lozenges (dequalinium chloride)
Eludril Mouthwash (chlorbutol, chlorhexidine gluconate)
Famel Pastilles (creosote, menthol)
Labosept Pastilles (dequalinium chloride)
Mentholatum Lozenges (amylmetacresol, eucalyptus oil, menthol)
Merocets Lozenges (cetylpyridinium chloride)
Mereothol Lozenges (cetylpyridinium chloride, cineole, menthol)
Merovit Lozenges (cetylpyridinium chloride, vitamin C)
Oraldene Solution (hexetidine)
Strepsils Original (amylmetacresol, dichlorobenzyl alcohol)
Strepsils with Vitamin C Lozenges (amylmetacresol dichlorobenzyl alcohol)
TCP Pastilles (phenol, halogenated phenol)
TCP Liquid (phenol, halogenated phenol)

Products with volatile oils and substances
Meggezones Pastilles (menthol)
Valda Pastilles (eucalyptus oil, menthol, thymol, guaiacol)

Stye

What is a stye and how should it be treated?

A stye or hordeolum is a boil at the root of an eyelash and is usually caused by a staphylococcal infection. The surrounding tissues may be inflamed and painful. The pocket of pus may sometimes be discharged by careful plucking of the affected lash with a pair of clean tweezers. Resolution is usually more rapid once the pus is cleared. The affected area may then be protected using an appropriate antiseptic eye ointment. Frequent recurrences will need to be referred to exclude more serious underlying problems such as diabetes.

Are other common conditions likely to be mistaken for styes?

Meibomian cysts may be confused with styes. In the former, however, the inflammation is further away from the lid margin and pain is minimal. The initial problem is due to blockage of the openings of the meibomian glands in the eye-lids but secondary infection of the cyst may give it a stye-like appearance. Meibomian cysts often need to be incised and curetted and referral is therefore required.

Precautions and when to refer

(R) Patients with recurrent styes (diabetics).

(R) If vision is impaired.

Product option

Brolene Eye Ointment (propamidine isethionate)

Sunburn

What are UVA and UVB rays?

The electromagnetic spectrum is shown in Figure 11. The rays responsible for suntan and sunburn fall in the ultraviolet region with wavelengths ranging from about 180–390 nm. This region is divided into three sub-regions referred to as UVA (320–390 nm), UVB (290–320 nm) and UVC (200–290) regions. UVC rays are effectively filtered off by the ozone layer of the stratosphere, UVB rays are the sunburn rays and UVA rays are normally the suntan rays. This UVA–UVB subdivision of ultraviolet rays is found useful by dermatologists because in addition to their relative effects on the suntanning process, some dermatological diseases react to one type of ray but not to the other.

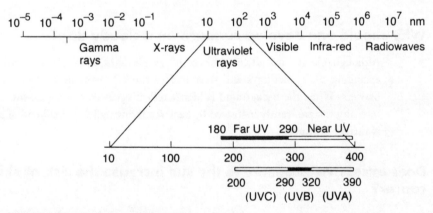

Fig. 11   The electromagnetic spectrum.

How does the skin normally protect itself against sunburn?

Sun protection is an adaptive process. On exposure to ultraviolet rays, the pigment cells of the skin (melanocytes) increase production of melanin which absorbs both UVA and UVB light. The effectiveness of melanin in preventing sunburn is evidenced by the fact that dark-skinned individuals are much less susceptible to the damaging effects of UV light than are light-skinned individuals. Substances other than melanin, such as urocanic acid, carotenoids, oxyhaemoglobin and reduced haemoglobin, may also add to the photoprotection provided by melanin but the effects are modest relative to those of melanin.

If melanin is an effective sunscreen agent why does sunburn develop?

The synthesis of melanin is a relatively slow process. The damage is already inflicted by the time adequate levels of melanin are produced to provide the necessary photoprotection. Such photoprotective responses are usually more useful for subsequent exposures to ultraviolet rays than for the initial exposure.

How do suntan agents work?

Three types of products are promoted as suntan agents. One type contains dihy-droxyacetone which reacts with skin to form a brownish colour. The colouring may provide protection against sunburn and lasts up to several weeks. A second type of product contain canthaxanthin, a carotenoid which colours the skin yellowish brown and therefore roughly mimics suntanning. The dye is toxic on the eye and should be avoided. A third type of product stimulates the melanocytes to increase melanin production. The products contain psoralens derived from citrus fruits, notably bergamot. These psoralens photobind to DNA and are therefore potentially damaging to the skin. Psoralens have generally been withdrawn although they were once popular in products such as Bergasol.

Why should one develop sunburn on a cloudy day?

Although clouds are efficient filters of visible light, they are less effective at excluding ultraviolet rays and over half of the UV light may cross thin cloud barriers. When the background is highly reflective, as on ski slopes, the UV light intensity is significantly increased by back scattering and the likelihood of sunburn is further enhanced.

Does excessive exposure to the sun increase the risk of skin cancer?

It is now generally accepted that excessive exposure to the sun does indeed increase the risk of skin cancer. Much of the supporting evidence comes from the high incidence of skin cancers among white settlers in countries such as Australia and South Africa. Increased exposure to the sun, coupled with fashions for more scanty clothing, has also been paralleled by an increase in the incidence of skin melanoma even in temperate climates. There is a particularly strong correlation between sunburn and skin melanoma.

Are there known risk factors to the development of skin cancer?

Generally, subjects who sunburn easily are more likely to develop skin cancer and subjects with lots of moles or with Celtic traits (blue eyes, fair or red hair and freckles) are at increased risk.

Does exposure to the sun cause skin ageing?

Evidence for the ageing effects of sun exposure is not difficult to obtain. The skins of Europeans migrating to warm sunny climates are generally more wrinkled than those of controls. Areas of the skin exposed to sunlight also generally show signs of ageing more obviously than areas normally covered by clothing. The explanation put forward for explaining the ageing effects of UV light is that of free radical-induced polymerization of skin proteins leading to loss of elasticity.

What changes accompany sunburn?

Erythema which is a manifestation of vasodilation in the superficial venous network, is the initial response to excessive exposure to ultraviolet rays. The erythema is accompanied by increased levels of prostaglandins in the affected area. The potent prostaglandin synthetase inhibitor, indomethacin, inhibits UVB and UVC erythema but not UVA erythema, thus indicating that different mechanisms must be operational. While other markers of inflammation, such as increased leucocyte migration, are also observed in sunburn, the extent of such changes is small relative to other types of inflammation.

The sunburnt skin becomes increasingly itchy and 2–8 hours after the onset of erythema, the skin starts to blister and the pain becomes intense. Clothing in contact with the naked skin becomes unbearable. The condition usually resolves itself over a period of about 10 days. In the presence of blisters, the protective barrier of the skin is disrupted and antiseptic cover may be required. Even in the absence of sunburn, biochemical changes are obvious and glucose-6-phosphate dehydrogenase activity increases in the epidermis while succinic dehydrogenase activity decreases. Skin thickening develops and the immune response is depressed. Langerhans cell alterations are also obvious.

Are phototoxic and photoallergenic reactions identical?

These terms are often used synonymously but they refer to sunlight-induced reactions with distinct mechanisms. Phototoxic reactions are exaggerated responses induced by the offending substances but for which no immunological basis can be identified. With such reactions there are clear dose–response relationships and when exposed to sufficiently high doses of the offending substances, most individuals will show a response. With photoallergenic responses, only a very small minority of those exposed to the offending substance will develop an adverse reaction, but once primed repeat exposures invariably initiate a response. Benoxaprofen, the antiarthritic drug which was withdrawn because of light hypersensitivity reactions, is an example of a drug showing phototoxicity. Sulphonamides and thiazides are thought to cause photoallergic reactions. In practice it is often difficult to dissociate phototoxic from photoallergenic reactions and the term photosensitivity is used to embrace both mechanisms of toxicity.

Is chronic use of sunscreen agents harmful?

There is little evidence that except for the rare hypersensitivity reactions, chronic use of sunscreen agents leads to adverse effects. Indeed for those exposed to strong sunlight in their daily occupations, chronic sunscreen use may reduce the risk of developing skin malignancies. One recent report indicates that chronic sunscreen use decreases circulating concentrations of 25–hydroxy vitamin D.

What substances are most commonly involved in photosensitivity reactions?

Both drugs and household chemicals are often involved in photosensitivity reactions. Some of the most commonly implicated are given in Table 21.

Modern sunbeds use UVA lamps. Are they completely safe?

UVA rays are certainly less harmful than UVB rays and therefore the modern suntanning lamps are safer than the old-fashioned UVA/UVB lamps. Excessive exposure to UVA lamps is, however, still unjustified since UVA light is known to enhance UVB damage, even after a lag time between the two exposures. Significantly also, most UVA lamps emit some UVB rays. Recent evidence suggests that continuous exposure to high doses of UVA light may be carcinogenic and cataracts may also develop on chronic exposure of the eye to intermittent UVA irradiation. UVA exposure is known to stimulate some phototoxic reactions and skin ageing is a predicted outcome. Adverse effects such as itching, nausea and skin rashes are common, particularly in women taking the contraceptive pill. For all these reasons, UVA sunlamps cannot be regarded as being completely safe.

Does frequent use of sunbed parlours predispose to fungal infections?

Cases of *tinea versicolor* have in fact been claimed to follow use of sunbeds. As with any public places, cross-infection by fungal diseases is enhanced. Some authors suggest that the humid environment and inadequate cleaning of sunbed areas increase the risk. Some experiments have shown that continued UV exposure depresses the immune response. Theoretically therefore, susceptibility to infection, including infection by fungi, may be enhanced.

How do sunscreen products work?

Sunscreen products contain two possible types of agents, opaque reflectant products and ultraviolet light-absorbing compounds. Compounds falling into the first group include various inert earths and pigments. Zinc oxide ointment, for example, is a widely used opaque sunscreen used by surfers. The ointments are cosmetically not very acceptable and UV absorbing formulations are usually preferred, particularly for products with medium to low sun-protection factors. Talc and titanium dioxide may be added to the high SPF formulations.

Table 21 Drugs and household chemicals implicated in photosensitivity reactions.

Acetohexamide	Flurouracil	Promethazine
Acridine dyes	Fluphenazine	Psoralens
Amiodarone	Frusemide (Furosemide)	Protriptyline
Amitriptyline	Glyseofulvin	Quinethazone
Anthracene	Gold salts	Retinoic acid
Bendrofluazide	Halogenated salicylanilides	Sodium aurothiomaleate
Benoxaprofen	Halogenated carbanilides	Sulphacytine
Benzthiazide	Halogenated phenols	Sulphamethazine
Bergamot oil	Haloperidol	Sulphamethizole
Bithionol	Hydrochlorothiazide	Sulphamethoxazole
Carbamazepine	Hydroflumethiazide	Sulfasalazine
Chlorothiazide	Imipramine	Sulphathiazole
Chlorpromazine	Metacycline	Sulphisoxazole
Chlorpheniramine	Methotrexate	Tetracycline
Chlorpropamide	Methoxpsoralen	Thioridazine
Chlortetracycline	Methylclothiazide	Tolazamide
Coal tar and derivatives	Musk ambrette	Tolbutamide
Contraceptive steroids	Metolazone	Trichlormethiazide
Cyclothiazide	Minocycline	Trifluoperazine
Cyproheptadine	Nalidixic acid	Trifluopromazine
Dacarbazine	Nortriptyline	Trimeprazine
Demeclocycline	Oxytetracycline	Trimethadione
Desipramine	Para-aminobenzoic acid	Trimipramine
Diphenhydramine	Para-amino acid esters	Trioxsalen
Disopyrimide	Perphenazine	Trisulphapyrimidines
Doxepine	Piperacetazine	Vinblastine
Doxycycline	Piroxicam	Wood tars
Eosin	Polythiazide	
Etratrinate	Prochlorperazine	

What types of compounds are the UV absorbing compounds?

Several series of compounds are widely used and these may be classified according to their screening efficiency in terms of ultraviolet light wavelengths. The narrow spectrum compounds screen out UVB rays and include para-aminobenzoic acid and its esters. These compounds have been associated with a relatively large number of photosensitivity reactions and may stain clothing on decomposition. The cinnamates, like most of the narrow spectrum sunscreens, are usually formulated with other more efficient compounds. Broader spectrum compounds include the benzophenones and derivatives of dibenzoylmethane. The benzophenones have absorption maxima in both the UVA and UVB regions and unlike many of the narrow spectrum compounds are highly photo-stable.

What is substantivity?

Substantivity is a term applied to topical agents, to describe the affinity of these agents to the skin. A highly substantive compound is one which remains on the skin despite prolonged exercise, sweating and exposure to water. Esters of para-aminobenzoic acid, for example, are highly substantive. So-called water-proof sunscreen agents are usually formulated with UV light-absorbing compounds of high substantivity. The formulation may also add to the substantivity of an active ingredient.

What is the SPF of a sunscreen agent?

SPF stands for sun protection factor, a numerical value representing the ratio of the time required to produce erythema in the presence of a sunscreen agent to the time required to produce the same end-point without the sunscreen. The technique used is not universal and the SPF factors of products made in different countries may not be directly comparable although more and more manufacturers are now adopting standardized techniques. Consistently however, the higher the SPF factor the greater the protection given by the sunscreen product. SPF values typically range from about 2 to 16. An SPF value of 16 generally refers to total block of UV rays.

Are the benefits to be derived from sunscreens with SPF values above 15 worthwhile?

Theoretically, the higher the SPF value, the greater the protection provided by the sunscreen agent. However, it has been argued that above an SPF of 15, there is little practical relevance to increases in SPF values. Some authorities are currently recommending that regulatory authorities maintain a maximum SPF of 20 based on the argument that no one gets exposed to sufficient ultraviolet radiation to require products with higher SPF values and there is little justification in unnecessarily exposing users to potentially toxic effects of high concentrations of chemicals.

Are there specific recommendations relating to sunscreens for specific skin types?

Skins are often categorized according to their susceptibility to the damaging effects of sunlight. Type I skin always burns easily without tanning. Type 2 skin burns easily with minimal tanning. Type III skin tans gradually but burns moderately. Type IV skin tans readily and rarely develops sunburn. Blue-eyed and fair-haired caucasians generally have Type I and II skins and for them, SPF factors of 7 or higher are required even under moderate sunlight exposure. Type IV skin usually does not need sunscreen protection under moderate exposures to normal temperature summer sunlight.

Are antihistamine compounds and local anaesthetic agents useful in sunburn?

In the presence of blistered skin both types of compounds will exert a beneficial antipruritic effect. However, both types of compounds are well known for their propensity to induce hypersensitivity reactions upon topical applications. Of the two groups, local anaesthetic agents would be the lesser of the two unattractive options.

Is Calamine Lotion useful in sunburn?

The phenolic content of the lotion will exert an antipruritic activity and the rapid aqueous evaporation may also produce a cooling anaesthetic effect. One potential problem is that calamine may cause granulomas if applied to broken skin. The lotion is therefore only suitable for non-blistered skin. This caution of course also applies to antihistaminic and local anaesthetic preparations containing suspended insoluble compounds (e.g. Caladryl Lotion).

How should sunburn be managed?

Mild sunburn is soothed by emollient lotions and creams. These may delay blistering and prevent skin infections. Antiseptic creams such as those containing chlorhexide may be useful when mild blistering is present. More serious sunburn will need referral.

What is the sunglasses syndrome?

This is a recently identified syndrome linked with the wearing of large sunglasses for prolonged periods of time. Patients complain of numbness and parasthesia over the cheeks and between the eyes. The symptoms gradually spread to affect the nose and upper incisors. The syndrome appears to be due to a compression neuropathy of the infra-orbital branch of the trigeminal nerve.

What advice should one give to those intending to sunbathe?

In addition to using a suitable sunscreen agent (re-applied every two to three hours when outdoors, even on a cloudy day) sunbathers should be advised to time and hence limit their exposure to the sun. They should avoid being sunburnt by making use of shaded areas and appropriate clothing once their timed exposures are exceeded. Wide broad-brimmed hats and sunglasses are recommended.

Precautions and when to refer_____

(R) When sunburn patients present with symptoms of systemic disturbance.

(R) If pre-existing dark wart-like lesions are activated (possible malignancy).

(!) Avoid topical antihistamines – may induce hypersensitivity reactions.

Product options

Sunblock or high SPF products
Piz Buin SPF 20 Sun Block Lotion (titanium dioxide, butylmethoxy-dibenzoylmethane, octyl methoxy-cinnamate)
Spectraban Lotion SPF 25 (para-aminobenzoic acid, padimate)
Spectraban Ultra Sunblock Lotion (titanium dioxide, padimate, oxybenzone, butylmethoxy-dibenzoyl-methane).
Sun E45 SPF 25 Sunblock Cream (zinc oxide, titanium dioxide)
Uvistat Babysun Sunblock Cream SPF22 (titanium dioxide, butylmethoxy-dibenzoylmethane, ethyl hexyl-p-methoxycinnamate)
Uvistat Lipscreen Ultrablock SPR 30 (titanium dioxide, butylmethoxy-dibenzoylmethane, methane benzylidene camphor)
Uvistat Long-Lasting Sun Cream SPF 25 (titanium dioxide, butylmethoxy-dibenzoylmethane)
Uvistat Sunblock Cream SPF 20 (titanium dioxide, butylmethoxy-dibenzoylmethane, ethyl hexyl-p-methoxycinnamate)

Mild sunburn products: Antiseptic anti-bacterial creams
Calamine Lotion BP
Lactocalamine Lotion (zinc oxide, phenol, witch hazel, zinc carbonate)
Solarcaine Cream (benzocaine, triclosan)
Solarcaine Lotion (benzocaine, triclosan)
Solarcaine Spray (benzocaine, triclosan)

Teeth

What causes dental caries?

Dental caries are usually caused by acid-producing bacteria present in the oral cavity. The bacteria, particularly *Streptococcus mutans* metabolize sucrose and other fermentable components of the diet to produce acids which dissolve enamel. The localized areas of demineralization on the tooth surface are then observed as dental caries. More rarely, tooth decay may be due to direct attack by acidic foods consumed, and in children tetracyclines may impair tooth formation to produce caries-like lesions.

What are gingivitis and periodontitis?

Soon after thorough tooth-brushing, a mucopolysaccharide film, including other adsorbed chemicals, is deposited on the tooth surface. This film provides an anchor for bacteria and current theory suggests that the initial invading bacteria are *Streptococcus sanguis* and gram positive rods. These bacteria form the basic plaque onto which *Streptococcus mutans* gain attachment eventually to become the predominant member of the plaque flora. Plaque, if not removed, progresses beyond the gingival margin to the underlying interfaces to induce inflammation of the gums, a condition generally referred to as gingivitis. Without appropriate treatment, the inflammation spreads into the deeper tissues leading to resorption of the alveolar bone and the tooth, being surrounded by a periodontal pocket teeming with bacteria, loses its stability. Gum disease which has progressed beyond gingivitis is referred to as periodontitis or more generally periodontal disease. Most authorities regard the latter as being the major threat to loss of teeth with ageing.

Why are some individuals more susceptible to caries than others?

Proper oral hygiene is an important preventative measure against caries. Clearly, those who are not careful about oral hygiene will develop more cavities than those who are. However, this parameter on its own does not fully explain the observed interindividual variations in the number of caries. There is a positive correlation between sugar intake and number of decayed teeth. A similar correlation exists between frequency of meals and number of caries. A hereditary influence is also shown in studies on monozygotic and dizygotic twins. Salivary gland disturbance and diseases such as Sjögren's syndrome may lead to rampant caries and it is known that deficiency in vitamins and minerals during dentition leads to an irreversible increase in susceptibility of the teeth to dental caries. Consumption of fluoride, a known protectant against caries, also shows wide variability. All these factors will therefore contribute to the observed inter-individual variability in the number of dental lesions.

How should dental and gum disease be prevented?

Regular thorough tooth-brushing is an essential requirement for optimum dental health. Avoidance of readily fermentable sugars is also important. Increasingly recognized is the need to maintain healthy gums and the use of dental floss ensures that dental plaque and food debris do not accumulated in the interdental spaces.

Does milk prevent tooth decay?

Milk is a source of calcium and fluoride ions which are essential for proper dentition and in the presence of deficiency states milk will clearly prevent tooth malformation. Whether this can be extrapolated to claiming that milk will prevent tooth decay under normal circumstances is debatable. It would be much more prudent to rely on alternative measures for maintaining dental health. Supplementary ingestion of skimmed milk is however unlikely to cause any harm.

Is fluoride supplementation useful in preventing tooth decay?

There is now little doubt that fluoride supplements are useful in preventing tooth decay in individuals receiving suboptimal levels of the element. While there is no consensus, most authorities support the use of fluoride supplements when drinking water provides less than 1 part per million of fluoride. Levels of 1.5 ppm, on the other hand, are generally regarded as adequate and higher levels are known to induce fluorosis, a condition characterized by discolouration, mottling and destruction of the tooth enamel.

How should fluoride supplements be administered?

A popular approach is fluoridation of water supplies. However, this approach is not always favoured and oral tablets or drops provide an alternative approach. Fluoride toothpastes and products for local application would clearly be ideal if effective. However, although they provide some protection, they are generally less effective than systemic supplementation because of poor bioavailability. However, some trials have shown comparable decreases in incidence of caries when topical and oral fluoride supplements were used. Some users would also prefer to trade off the potentially poorer activity of topical products against any potential systemic adverse effects which may accompany oral supplementation.

How do fluoride ions protect teeth against decay?

Surprisingly, the exact mechanism is not known but published data suggest that fluoride, through an effect on crystallinity, surface morphology and carbonate-content of hydroxyapatite, decreases the dissolution rate of the enamel in acidic conditions thereby making carious lesions less likely.

Are antimicrobial agents useful for the control of caries?

In the absence of *Streptococcus mutans*, caries are much less likely to develop and indeed, in the absence of buccal bacteria, caries do not appear in spite of a sugar-rich diet. Therefore, control of aciduric bacteria by antimicrobial agents is an attractive approach to preserving dental health. However, a sterile buccal cavity is not a realistic target and it is as yet unclear how commonly-used oral antiseptics affect the buccal microflora in the long term. Much of the microbiological work on the control of dental caries has therefore focused on controlling the density of buccal bacteria or more specifically on reducing the density of *S. Mutans*.

Antiseptic mouthwashes reduce salivary bacterial counts but these rapidly rise to pre-wash levels so that any protection derived from the mouthwashes is transient. The best methods for caries control so far appears to be avoidance of sugar and proper dental hygiene based largely on thorough physical cleaning of the teeth. For certain groups of patients, such as the handicapped, an antimicrobial product may be a necessary adjunct to dental health. If a mouthwash or other topical product is recommended then a chlorhexidine-based product would be preferable to a phenol-based or a quaternary ammonium-based product, although triclosan appears to be a promising new candidate in more recent trials.

How often should dental checks be carried out?

The dental profession usually recommends twice yearly checks. A recent review of the claimed advantages of the 6-monthly checks found little justification for them and the recommendation made was that routine dental checks could be reduced to an annual visit. Part of the justification is that dental health has been steadily improving over the past 15 years and the need for dental fillings of minor lesions is now less clear given our better understanding of spontaneous remineralization and healing of these lesions.

Which sugars are cariogenic and which are not?

Sucrose, maltose, lactose, glucose and fructose are all cariogenic, particularly when consumed as solids. Foods high in starch and low in dissacharides, but not free from sucrose, may lead to more prolonged lowering in plaque pH than sucrose-rich food and could therefore be highly cariogenic. Polyols such as mannitol, sorbitol, maltitol and xylitol are essentially non-cariogenic. Lycasin, consisting of a series of slow fermenting saccharides, particularly sorbitol, is an increasingly widely used sweetening agent in the so-called sugar-free formulations for paediatric use. Sorbose, chlorosorbose and non-nutritive sweeteners such as acesulfame, saccharin and aspartame are also safe for teeth.

Do sugar-free formulations therefore help in reducing dental caries?

While, intuitively, sugar-free formulations would appear worthwhile, the supporting evidence is equivocal except for medications administered on a chronic basis at high dose frequenceis to patients who are not able to look after their teeth. Patients with cystic fibrosis, for example, receive prophylactic antibiotics on a chronic basis. Physically handicapped patients form another vulnerable group who may benefit from sugar-free formulations. For the short-term treatment of self-limiting conditions, sugar-free formulations are less worthwhile.

Does infant-feeding on demand increase the incidence of dental decay?

The adverse effects of constant sucking of soothers dipped in syrupy products on dental health is well known. More recently a number of reports have drawn attention to similar dangers associated with constant sucking of milk from a bottle or constant breast feeding during the night. The constant exposure of the teeth to sucrose or lactose is thought to be responsible for the observed aggravation of dental decay in such infants. To reduce such problems a modified fixed time feeding schedule may be preferable or alternatively a short feed with water after each milk feed may be helpful. In practice these suggestions are extremely hard to adopt.

Can drugs induce dental problems?

The role of tetracycline in damaging erupting teeth has already been mentioned. Gum hyperplasia arising from phenytoin ingestion is well recognized. More recently nifedipine has been reported to be associated with the same problem. Drugs with anticholinergic adverse effects which interfere with normal salivation may interfere with the normal cleansing and self-protection of the buccal cavity thereby making caries more likely. For patients receiving such drugs, advice to increase mouth rinsing during the day may be beneficial. Corrosive drugs should not be placed next to the tooth and the previously common practice of placing aspirin tablets next to teeth for the control of dental pain should now be abandoned.

Are vaccines against dental caries likely?

If the microbial aetiology of dental caries is correct and the offending bacterium is *S. mutans* then it should theoretically be possible to develop a vaccine against the disease. The problem would be much more difficult if many different microorganisms were involved. Much research effort is already directed at designing a safe anti-decay vaccine and although antigens derived from *S. mutans* have been shown to protect experimental animals against caries, cross-reactivity of the antigens with heart and muscle tissues remains a major concern. The safety of any proposed vaccine against caries therefore needs to be fully established and this is likely to take a few years yet. It is interesting to note that some authors in fact are of the opinion that improving dental health in the developed countries is due more to acquired immunity than to fluoride, dental treatment or changes in sugar consumption. Tooth brushing, it is suggested, produces a massive immunological challenge as the bristles abrade the mucous membranes in contact with the offending micro-organisms.

What is the cause of teething problems in infants?

Pharmacists and other health care professionals are often asked to recommend something for 'teething' and in many cases the automatic reaction is to advise the use of a teething gel or an analgesic suspension. Such an approach is not sound as so called 'teething' problems are not always associated with pain and the use of anaesthetic or analgesic compounds without due cause is unwarranted. There is also no demonstrable association between the eruption of teeth and sleeplessness, fever, rashes, diarrhoea or infections and the use of combination teething mixtures containing sedative antihistamines is also not justified. In most cases when advice is sought for teething problems, reassurance is all that is needed. When signs of systematic problems such as pyrexia, diarrhoea and convulsions are described a thorough investigation is required and self-treatment is not advised.

Are teething gels safe to use?

Occasionally, a case can be made for the use of a teething gel and with careful use there is little danger of any harm arising from such use except for the rare cases of hypersensitivity to the local anaesthetic or excipient present in the formulations. More recently, some questions have been raised about the possible implications of the salicylate content of some of the teething gels (Bonjela and Teegel). The amount of salicylate absorbed from application of the teething gels is likely to be small and the cause and effect relationship between Reye's syndrome and salicylate ingestion is by no means established. Based on these facts, many authorities, including a number of drug regulatory authorities, do not contraindicate the use of those gels. However, given the mythical nature of most cases of teething problems, until the issue is completely resolved there is little justification for unnecessarily exposing the infant to medication that is not needed.

Are denture adhesives safe?

Denture adhesives, either in paste or powder form, are often useful in providing added confidence to denture wearers. However, well-fitting dentures do not require adhesives to remain in place. Prolonged use may promote use beyond the time when readjustments are required and damage to oral structures may ensue. Without regular thorough cleansing of the dentures, the adhesives may also serve as a growth medium for micro-organisms leading to bad breath and oral infections. The occasional hypersensitivity reactions to denture adhesives are also known to occur.

How safe are denture liners and cushions?

There is now little justification for the use of these denture aids as long-term use may lead to faster bone loss, continuing irritation and sores.

How should dentures be cleaned?

Recent evidence suggests that overnight soaking in an alkaline peroxide solution may be more effective than brushing. However, a combination of the two methods may be preferable as brushing will remove the larger pieces of entrapped debris while soaking will help to sterilize and dislodge invisible plaque. At least once daily is recommended and thorough rinsing prior to insertion into the mouth is important.

Are disclosing tablets useful?

Disclosing agents help reveal plaque deposits and are helpful in ensuring proper tooth brushing. However, once a proper tooth brushing technique is established the use of disclosing tablets is probably unnecessary.

Are formulae against sensitive teeth effective?

Dentine hypersensitivity is a condition characterized by pain whenever the affected tooth is exposed to thermal, chemical or mechanical stimuli. The aetiology of the condition is poorly defined but one popular theory is that unmyelinated nerve endings in the most pulpal part of dentine and afferent nerves in the peripheral pulp provide the morphological basis for the problem. Treatment with strontium chloride, formaldehyde, resins, silver nitrate and potassium hydroxide have all been reported to provide symptomatic relief but little formulation optimization work has been reported in the literature.

Are natural products useful in preventing dental caries?

Natural products are currently attracting much consumer and scientific interest and in the field of oral hygiene, sanguinarine is at the centre of that interest. Sanguinarine is a benzophenantridinium alkaloid obtained from the rhizome of *Sanguinaria canadensis* (Sanguinaria). Sanguinaria extracts have been used as a herbal remedy in North America for more than a century but the current focus is on their anti-plaque and anti-caries activities which are probably due to an anti-microbial effect. Observed clinical effects have however, so far, been conflicting.

What causes toothache?

Toothache is caused by exposure of dental free-nerve endings as a result of breakdown of the protective enamel on the tooth. Toothache therefore follows dental decay. Often, infection of the underlying tissues sets in and pain intensifies.

Precautions and when to refer_____

(R) Toothache with obvious inflammation, abscess or fever should be referred immediately.

(!) Clove oil and tooth tinctures may damage nerves.

(!) See under analgesics if analgesics recommended.

(!) Excessive fluoride intake may cause mottling of teeth.

Product options for toothache_____

Oral analgesics   Clove oil

Thrush

What causes vaginal thrush?

Thrush is a yeast infection of the lower female genital tract. Presenting symptoms include vaginal discharge and soreness around the introitus. Contamination of the vaginal area by *candida albicans* present round the perineum is a common cause of the infection. This risk may be increased by minor trauma during sexual intercourse. True sexual transmission by an infected but asymptomatic partner may also occur. Thrush may also be more likely during pregnancy possibly due to depressed immunity.

What is oral thrush?

Oral thrush is a yeast infection of the oral cavity. The same organisms seen in genital thrush are involved. Nystatin lozenges are the most widely prescribed therapy for oral thrush. Gentian violet paint, once widely prescribed for oral thrush, is now contraindicated because of its known cytotoxicity. Non-prescription remedies for oral thrush are not very effective although polynoxylin lozenges and quaternary ammonium chloride (e.g. dequalinium) lozenges may be of occasional use.

How should vaginal thrush be treated?

Since the infection is fungal in origin, antifungal therapy is the most effective. Three imidazole agents, clotrimazole, miconazole and econazole, are now available as intravaginal creams and pessaries for self-medication. Single dose therapy with the appropriate formulation is as effective as multiple-dose therapy. Moreover single dose therapy benefits from convenience and hence improved compliance. Douches, acidifying pessaries and lactobacillus preparations have their proponents but none of them is consistently effective. Gentian violet paint may be cytotoxic and is now contraindicated. Povidone-iodine is less effective than the imidazole pessaries and may also be more hazardous as a result of a partial absorption of iodine into the systemic circulation.

How do the imidazole agents work?

The imidazole agents inhibit ergosterol and fatty acid synthesis by the yeasts. This leads to increased membrane permeability, uncontrolled cell wall synthesis and cell death. Since only the unionized weakly basic imidazole molecule is active, concurrent use of acidifying agents should be avoided.

What problems are associated with the intravaginal formulations?

Contact between contraceptive diaphragms or sheaths and the soft vaginal pessaries or creams may damage the contraceptive barriers.

Some 10% of an intravaginal dose of the antifungal imidazole agents are absorbed into the systemic circulation. Therefore patients who previously have reacted adversely to oral imidazoles should avoid their intravaginal use also.

What predisposes to vaginal candidiasis?

Predisposing factors include:

- pregnancy
- use of the contraceptive pill
- minor trauma during intercourse
- wearing of tight, occlusive underwear
- diabetes mellitus
- use of irritant applications
- antibiotic and cytotoxic therapy
- oral steroid therapy
- iron and zinc deficiency.

When should patients with vaginal candidiasis be referred?

Referral by the pharmacist to the doctor is recommended if the patient:

- has had similar infections more than twice in the previous six months
- has a history of sexually transmitted disease
- is pregnant
- is under 16 or over 60 years of age
- has abnormal vaginal bleeding or blood-stained discharge
- has dysuria or pain in the lower abdomen
- has any vulval or vaginal blisters, ulcers or sores
- has had a reaction to a previous course of treatment for vaginal candidiasis
- is suffering from the infection for the first time.

Product options

First-line agents: Vaginal thrush
Canesten 1 Vaginal Tablet (clotrimazole)
Canesten 10% VC Vaginal Cream
   (clotrimazole)
Canesten Combi (pessary plus vulval
   cream, clotrimazole)
Deflucan One Capsule (fluconazole)
Ecostatin Pessaries (econazole)
Ecostatin 1 Pessary (econazole)
Ecostatin Twinpack (pessary + vulval
   cream, econazole)

Frereron Soft Pessary (miconazole)
Gyno-Daktarin Ovule (micronazole)
Gyno-Pevaryl Pessaries (econazole)
Gyno-Pevaryl 1 Pessary (econazole)
Gyno-Pevaryl Combipack (econazole)
Gyno-Pevaryl CP Pack (econazole pessary
   + vulval cream)
Tavogyn Vaginal Tablets (isoconazole)

First-line agents: Oral thrush
Daktarin Oral Gel (miconazole)

Second-line products (lengthy treatment regimes)
Canesten Vaginal Cream (clotrimazole)
Gyno-Daktarin Intravaginal Cream
   (miconazole)

Gyno-Daktarin Pessaries (miconazole)
Gyno-Pevaryl Cream (econazole)

Non-specific products
Aci-Jel Vaginal Jelly (buffered acetate)

Travel sickness

What causes travel sickness?

Travel sickness is induced by repetitive motion. The most widely accepted theory, known as the 'conflict theory' suggests that motion sickness arises because of a mismatch in the information reaching the brain from the vestibular system (Figure 12), the eyes and the non-vestibular proprioceptors. Russian scientists on the other hand seem to prefer the 'cephalid-fluid shift theory' which proposes that motion induces haemodynamic alterations, leading to hypoxia and hence symptoms of travel sickness.

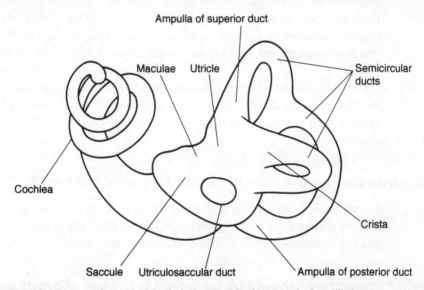

Fig. 12 The membraneous labyrinth, involved in the control of equilibrium.

What are the symptoms of travel sickness?

Travel sickness is characterized by nausea, pallor, unease, cold sweating and in severe cases, vomiting. The symptoms may be present independently or simultaneously.

How do travel sickness remedies work?

The available and proven medications for travel sickness fall into two distinct groups, those that exert an anticholinergic effect on central nervous system receptors and those that activate the central sympathetic areas. It has been suggested that antihistamines probably work through their anticholinergic side-effects.

Which is the best remedy for travel sickness?

Hyoscine is probably the most effective agent against travel sickness. However, the drug appears to have a narrow therapeutic window and adverse effects including blurred vision and confusion have been reported even with therapeutic doses. Controlled delivery, with a transdermal patch, reduces the likelihood of adverse effects but these are not eliminated. The drug is useful for short journeys when the risk of drug accumulation is minimized.

Of the antihistamines, cyclizine is a good choice but its central excitatory effects have led to abuse. Meclizine (meclozine) is effective on a once daily dosage and is very similar to cyclizine in activity profile. Cinnarizine is a widely promoted antihistamine but clinical superiority over other antihistamines has not been demonstrated. Its use has been marred by reports of extrapyramidal side-effects. Dimenhydrinate is the theoclate salt of diphenhydramine, a relatively strong sedative antihistamine. Data on its efficacy in travel sickness is sparse. Promethazine is also sedative and is widely used in the United Kingdom for the paediatric population.

For adults on short journeys, hyoscine may be the best choice. Meclizine and cyclizine are useful alternatives for longer journeys unless a transdermal hyoscine patch is used. Promethazine elixir is probably the product of first choice for children.

Is it true that ginger may be useful for travel sickness?

A small study indicated that ginger was indeed effective in reducing symptoms; however this needs to be confirmed. A possible mode of action is counter-stimulation thus detracting from the effects of nauseous stimulation.

What precautions should be observed in the use of drugs against motion sickness?

All of the drugs commonly used exert significant anticholinergic effects. The most potent in this respect are hyoscine, cyclizine and meclizine. Their use should therefore be avoided in patients with glaucoma, prostate enlargement or urinary retention. Use of drugs should of course be ideally avoided during pregnancy. In this respect, meclizine, cyclizine and dicyclomine have all, at some time, been claimed to induce foetal malformations. The elderly and those with central nervous diseases should probably ideally avoid the potent anticholinergics. The potential targets for side-effects of the anticholinergic compounds are shown in Figure 13.

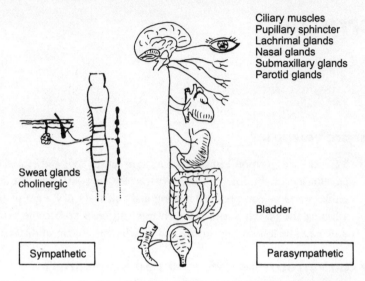

Ciliary muscles
Pupillary sphincter
Lachrimal glands
Nasal glands
Submaxillary glands
Parotid glands

Sweat glands
cholinergic

Bladder

Sympathetic

Parasympathetic

Fig. 13   Target sites for side-effects of anticholinergic drugs such as hyoscine.

Precautions and when to refer

(!) Avoid hyoscine, cyclizine and meclizine in glaucoma, prostate enlargement or urinary retention, the elderly, the very young and CNS disease.

(!) Avoid diphenhydramine, dimenhydrinate, cyclizine, dicyclomine and meclozine in pregnancy.

(!) Avoid hyoscine, cyclizine and meclozine in the elderly and the very young.

(!) Avoid hyoscine in acute porphyria.

Product options

Avomine Tablets (promethazine theoclate)
Dramamine Tablets (dimenhydrinate)
Joy-Rides Tablets (hyoscine hydrobromide)
Junior Kwells Tablets (hyoscine
   hydrobromide)
Kwells Tablets (hyoscine hydrobromide)
Phenergan Syrup (promethazine
   hydrochloride)

Q-Mazine Syrup (promethazine
   hydrochloride)
Sea-legs Tablets (meclozine hydrochloride)
Stugeron Tablets (cinnarizine)
Valoid Tablets (cyclizine hydrochloride)

Verrucae

What are verrucae?

Verrucae are common benign tumours seen on the foot and caused by the human papillomavirus. In other words, verrucae are warts affecting the foot. However, unlike warts in non-pressure bearing and relatively dry areas of the skin, those affecting the plantar surface may enlarge and crack to become highly painful on walking. The lesions vary in size and may be up to 2 cm in diameter.

How can verrucae be differentiated from corns?

Corns are particularly painful when direct pressure is applied to them whereas verrucae are painful when lateral pressure is applied. Verrucae may also be painful even without application of pressure whereas corns are usually painless in the absence of physical contact. Verrucae most commonly affect the young while corns affect adults predominantly, although ill-fitting shoes may induce corn formation even in children. Involvement of the blood vessels leads to rapid visualization of bleeding points within the growth in verrucae. No such vessels are visible in corns. A clinical history will also suggest a sudden onset for verrucae and a slow progression for corns. However, slow enlargement of verrucae may give the impression of slow progression before treatment or advice is sought. Corns are usually hard and glassy in appearance whereas verrucae are usually soft and spongy.

How should verrucae be treated?

Keratolytic preparations (salicylic acid and lactic acid) are useful first-line treatments. More persistent warts may require formaldehyde foot baths or formaldehyde or gluteraldehyde lotions and gels. Both aldehydes may cause sensitization. Podophyllin products are still used but are no longer recommended. Cryotherapy may be required for recalcitrant cases.

Precautions and when to refer

(R) Diabetic patients.

(R) Lesions not on the plantar surface.

(R) Lesions not improving after 8 weeks.

Lesions which bleed or change colour.

 Recommend avoidance of walking barefoot in communal areas.

Product options

Salicylic-acid-based products

Salicylic acid collodion BP

Bazuka Gel (salicylic acid, lactic acid)

Carnation Verruca Treatment (salicylic acid)

Compound W Plasters and Liquid (salicylic acid)

Cuplex Gel (salicylic acid, copper acetate)

Duofilm Paint (salicylic acid, lactic acid)

Occlusal Application (salicylic acid)

Salatac Gel (salicylic acid, lactic acid)

Salactol Paint (salicylic acid, lactic acid)

Scholl Verruca Removal System (salicylic acid)

Verrugon Ointment (salicylic acid)

Glutaraldehyde-containing products

Glutarol (glutaraldehyde)

Verucasep Gel (glutaraldehyde)

Podophyllum-based products (contra-indicated in pregnancy)

Posafilin Ointment (podophyllum resin, salicylic acid)

Vitamins and dietary supplements

What are vitamins and how many are there?

Vitamins are organic substances which are required in small amounts for the maintenance of health but which cannot be manufactured by the cells of the body. To date only 13 substances are generally regarded as vitamins (Table 22). Four of the vitamins are oil-soluble and the other nine are water-soluble.

Some substances which are sometimes called vitamins but are not generally regarded as such are shown in Table 23.

Table 22 Substances known as vitamins, their common synonyms and some biological functions.

Vitamins	Common synonyms	Some biological functions, mainly through co-enzymic action
A	Retinol	Vision, epithelial regeneration
B_1	Aneurine Thiamine	Amino acid metabolism
B_2	Riboflavin	Fat metabolism; oxidation
B_5	Pantothenic acid	Carbohydrate and fat metabolism
B_6	Pyridoxine	Amino acid and protein metabolism
B_{12}	Cyanocobalamin	Replication of genes, red blood cell formation
C	Ascorbic acid	Collagen synthesis
D	Calciferol Cholecalciferol	Calcium metabolism and bone formation
E	Alpha tocopherol	Neurological function, cell integrity; antioxidant
Folic acid	Folacin	Purine and thymine synthesis for DNA
H	Biotin	Carbohydrate, amino acid metabolism
K	Menaphthone	Blood clotting mechanism
Niacin	Nicotinic acid	Oxidation and energy transfer

Table 23 Some substances occasionally claimed to be vitamins but not generally recognized as such.

Vitamin B_4	6–Aminopurine
Vitamin B_{15}	Pangamic acid
Vitamin B_{13}	Orotic acid
Vitamin B_{14}	Xanthopterin
Vitamin B_{17}	Laetrile
Vitamin B_T	Carnitine
Bios I	Inositol
Vitamin F	Mixture of unsaturated fatty acids (linoleic, linolenic, arachidonic)
Vitamin H	Biotin
Vitamin L	0–Aminobenzoic acid
Vitamin T	Tegotin
Vitamin U	Methylmethioninesulphonium chloride
Ubiquinone	

How much of each vitamin do we need to stay healthy?

There is no simple answer to this question as requirements will depend among others on age, current metabolic state and extent of physical activity. Additionally, with most vitamins, deficiency is difficult to induce and therefore basal requirements cannot be calculated. For this reason one considers recommended daily allowances rather than strict requirements. Current allowances recommended by British authorities are listed in Table 24. These do not necessarily coincide with allowances recommended by other health authorities. Note that allowances are not recommended for some of the vitamins.

What are the main dietary sources of the vitamins?

A normal diet usually meets the vitamin requirements of the body. Only when there are extremes of food faddism or food deprivation does deficiency become apparent. At risk groups include strict vegetarians, the elderly and some immigrant groups. Table 25 lists some major dietary sources of the vitamins.

Can large doses of vitamins help prevent or cure diseases?

There are cases of inborn errors of metabolism which lead to inefficient use of vitamins. Examples are pyrdoxine dependency states due to abnormality in glutamic acid decarboxylase and kynureninase and increased biotin requirements due to deficiency of 3-methycrotonyl CoA carboxylase. In these rare cases, use of vitamin doses well above the recommended daily allowances are acceptable and

Table 24 Recommended daily amounts of some vitamins for male and female popoulation groups in the United Kingdom (*Dietary Reference Values fod Food Energy and Nutrients for the United Kingdom*, HMSO Press. Reproduced with the permission of the Controller of HMSO).

Age	Thiamine	Riboflavin	Niacin (nicotinic acid equivalent)	Vitamin B₆	Vitamin B₁₂	Folate	Vitamin C	Vitamin A	Vitamin D
	mg	mg	mg	mg†	µg	µg	mg	µg	µg
0–3 months	0.2	0.4	3	0.2	0.3	50	25	350	8.5
4–6 months	0.2	0.4	3	0.2	0.3	50	25	350	8.5
7–9 months	0.2	0.4	4	0.3	0.4	50	25	350	7
10–12 months	0.3	0.4	5	0.4	0.4	50	25	350	7
1–3 years	0.5	0.6	8	0.7	0.5	70	30	400	7
4–6 years	0.7	0.8	11	0.9	0.8	100	30	500	—
7–10 years	0.7	1.0	12	1.0	1.0	150	30	500	—
Males									
11–14 years	0.9	1.2	15	1.2	1.2	200	35	600	—
15–18 years	1.1	1.3	18	1.5	1.5	200	40	700	—
19–50 years	1.0	1.3	17	1.4	1.5	200	40	700	—
50+ years	0.9	1.3	16	1.4	1.5	200	40	700	**
Females									
11–14 years	0.7	1.1	12	1.0	1.2	200	35	600	—
15–18 years	0.8	1.1	14	1.2	1.5	200	40	600	—
19–50 years	0.8	1.1	13	1.2	1.5	200	40	600	—
50+ years	0.8	1.1	12	1.2	1.5	200	40	600	**
Pregnancy	0.1***	+0.3	*	*	*	+100	+10	+100	10
Lactation:									
0–4 months	+0.2	+0.5	+2	*	+0.5	+ 60	+30	+350	10
4+ months	+0.2	+0.5	+2	*	+05	+ 60	+30	+350	10

*No increment   ** After age 65 the RNI is 10µg for men and women   *** For last trimester only   † Based on protein providing 14.7 per cent of EAR for energy

Table 25   Some dietary sources of the recognized vitamins.

Vitamin A or its products	Fish liver oil, fortified margarine, butter, eggs, carrots.
Vitamin B_1	Yeast, wheat germ and fortified foods such as breakfast cereals and bread, wholemeal flour, beans, cheese, all leafy vegetables.
Vitamin B_6	Eggs, fish, wholemeal flour, vegetables.
Vitamin B_{12}	Food of animal origin (liver, kidney, lean meat, fish, eggs).
Vitamin C	Citrus fruits, tomatoes, green vegetables.
Vitamin D	Fish liver oil, fortified margarine, butter, cheese, eggs, milk.
Vitamin E	Nuts, vegetables, dairy products.
Vitamin K	Liver, lean meat, spinach, broccoli, green cabbage, turnip greens, lettuce.
Folic acid	Green-leaved vegetables, liver, kidney.
Pantothenic acid	Yeast, liver, eggs.
Nicotinic acid	Meat, fish, wheat flour.
Biotin	Yeast, liver, kidney, milk.

indeed required. Much less well accepted is the use of megadoses of vitamins for a variety of conditions including premenstrual tension, cancer, rheumatism, impotence and side-effects of the contraceptive pill. Table 26 lists some of the acceptable, controversial and unacceptable uses of vitamins above the recommended daily allowances. In some instances, such as in the prevention of blindness and osteoporosis, the large doses are used only at intervals for practical reasons.

Is it true that vitamins can boost children's intelligence quotients?

It is certainly to be expected that deficiency in vitamins, which are necessary for metabolism, will impair both physical and intellectual performances. Therefore it is not surprising that claims are often made that vitamins improve the IQ, particularly in children. There is some evidence to suggest that vitamin supplements may indeed improve the IQs of children on deficient diets. However, the trials conducted so far have been flawed by poor statistical design and conflicting results have been reported. Much more work is necessary before a valid claim can be made.

Are the vitamins potentially toxic?

There is little doubt that excessive doses of the oil-soluble vitamins are toxic. Vitamin A and D toxicity leading to liver disease, metastic calcification and renal problems are well known examples. At one time, a common view was that water-soluble vitamins were unlikely to be toxic since any excess is rapidly excreted in the urine. This view is now known to be erroneous and hepatoxicity, alopecia and

Table 26 Use of vitamins at doses well above the recommended daily allowance.

Vitamin	Acceptable	Controversial	Condemned
Vitamin A	Prevention of blindness at twice yearly dosing	Reduction of cancer risk	
	Analogues for acne		Vitamin A for acne
Vitamin B_1 (Thiamine)	Wernicke's encephalopathy Beri Beri Heart disease		
Vitamin B_6 (pyridoxine)	Infantile convulsive disorders Urinary oxalate stones	Premenstrual tension Oral contraceptives Menopause Carpal tunnel syndrome	
Vitamin C		Common cold	
Vitamin D		Osteoporosis	
Vitamin E		Intermittent claudication Postoperative embolism	Sex function Prevention of heart disease
Pantothenic acid		Rheumatoid arthritis	
Nicotinic acid	Hartnup disease	Hyperlipidaemia	Psychiatric disease
Multivitamins		Neural tube defects	Hangover Brain dysfunction
Vitamins in general	Specific inherited metabolic disorders Malabsorption syndromes		
Folic acid	Prevention of side-effects of anti-cancer drugs	Cervical dysplasia	

arrythmias following excessive niacin intake and peripheral neuropathy following pyridoxine abuse have been described in the literature. Table 27 lists some of the potentially toxic reactions. The consensus, however, is that at doses of vitamins ranging up to 200% of the recommended daily allowances, toxicity is highly unlikely.

Table 27 Potential toxicity of excessive doses of vitamins and elemental supplements.

Vitamin	Toxic effects
Vitamin A	Teratogenicity Hair loss Raised intracranial pressure Hepatotoxicity Ingrown toenials Skin abnormalities, including dryness and itchiness
Vitamin B$_3$ (niacin, nicotinamide)	Hair loss Arrhythmias Hepatotoxicity Peptic ulcers Hypotension
Vitamin B$_6$ (pyridoxine)	Peripheral sensory neuropathy Interference with action of levodopa
Vitamin C (ascorbic acid)	Renal stones in individuals with cystinuria, oxalosis and hyperuricaemia
Vitamin D	Hypercalcaemia Renal calcinonis Hypertension
Vitamin E	Increased warfarin effects
Vitamin K	Haemolytic anaemia Neonatal jaundice Depressed warfarin effects

Do some drugs interfere with vitamin utilization and if so can the reverse also take place?

Both types of interaction are known to occur. Pyridoxine, for example, decreases the therapeutic effect of levodopa and vitamin K interferes with warfarin action, while anticonvulsants increase the requirements for vitamin D. In all the cases where vitamin requirements are increased by concomitant drug ingestion, the value of vitamin supplements is still uncertain. Table 28 lists some of the reported drug–vitamin interactions.

How important are iron and vitamin supplements in pregnancy?

Iron and folic acid supplements are widely given to pregnant women based on the knowledge that during pregnancy red-cell mass increases by about 25% and folate requirements increase in line. This practice has been challenged largely on the basis of economic waste. More recently however, the Department of Health in the UK has recommended that women planning a pregnancy should increase their folic acid intake by 400 µg daily. This advice This advice follows on from epidemiological evidence showing than an adequate folic acid intake from conception until the 12th

Table 28 Drugs which have been reported to increase vitamin requirements or reduce their availability.

Vitamin A	Spironolactone, liquid praffin, cholestryamine, neomycin
Folic acid	Oral contraceptives, anticonvulsants, methotrexate, pyrimethamine, co-trimoxazole, trimethoprim, triamterene, cycloserine, sulphasalazine (axulfidine)
Vitamin B_{12}	Biguanides (metformin and phenformin), anticonvulsants, oral contraceptives, cholestyramine, neomycin, colchicine, para-aminosalicylate (PAS)
Vitamin B_6	Isoniazid, penicillamine, levodopa hydrallazine, oral contraceptives, alcohol
Nicotinic acid	Isoniazid
Vitamin D	Anticonvulsants
Vitamin K	Anticonvulsants, antibiotics, liquid paraffin, vitamin A, sulphonamides, cholestyramine, neomycin
Vitamin C	Aspirin, oral contraceptives, steroids, barbiturates, tetracycline

week of pregnancy reduces the risk of neural tube defects – spina bifida, anencephaly and encephalocele. Women with a previous history of newborns with neural tube defects may reduce the risk of recurrence by taking 4 mg folic acid daily. Women on anticonvulsants are at increased risk of being folate deficient and would require specialist advice.

When should advice about increasing folate intake be given?

The earlier the advice is given the better since after 12 weeks of conception, it is probably too late. Therefore some form of targeting potential mothers with appropriate information during their visits to the pharmacy would be invaluable.

Can the additional folate required be obtained from the diet?

Supplements are the most reliable method for ensuring an adequate dose. However, it is possible to obtain 400 µg of folate from a well-balanced diet. A helping of fortified cereal will provide some 100 µg. A serving of brussel sprouts, spring greens, broccoli, green beans and spinach will provide another 50 µg. Potatoes, most other fresh vegetables, fresh fruit, nuts, baked beans, bread, milk, salmon, beef and orange juice also contain at last 15 µg of folate per serving.

Should folic acid be recommended during pregnancy?

The official Department of Health (UK) recommendation is that all women planning a pregnancy should take a daily dietary supplement of 0.4 mg of folic acid. For women with a history of bearing a child with a neural tube defect, the recommended dose is 4 milligrams daily. The supplements should be continued through to the twelfth week of pregnancy. For those unwilling to take supplements, the list of foods rich in folic acid in Table 29 may be useful.

What are the essential trace elements?

The nine trace elements, chromium, cobalt, copper, iodine, iron, manganese, molybdenum, selenium and zinc, known to be essential to man, are called the essential trace elements. A further six, arsenic, fluoride, nickel, silicon, tin and vanadium are thought to be essential to other mammals. Of the latter six, only fluoride has a well-established function in man, namely maintenance of dental structure. Tables 30 and 31 list the UK recommended intakes for various minerals and trace elements, reprinted with the permission of HMSO.

Table 29   Foods rich in folic acid.

	Micrograms (per typical serving)
Boiled vegetables	
Broccoli	30
Brussels sprouts	100
Cabbage	25
Cauliflower	45
Green beans	50
Peas	30
Potatoes old	45
Potatoes new	40
Spinach	80
Fruit	
Grapefruit	20
Orange	50
Orange juice	40
Cereals and cereal products	
White bread, average (2 slices)	25
Wholemeal bread, average (2 slices)	40
Soft grain bread (fortified with folic acid)	105
Cornflakes (fortified with folic acid)	100
Branflakes (unfortified)	40
Branflakes (fortified with folic acid)	100
Other foods	
Bovril (per cup)	95
Yeast extract (on bread)	40
Milk, whole/semi-skimmed (one pint)	35

Table 30(a) Recommended daily amounts of some minerals for male and female population groups in the United Kingdom (*Dietary Reference Values for Food Energy and Nutrients for the United Kingdom*, HMSO Press; reproduced with the permission of the Controller of HMSO.).

Age	Calcium[1] mmol	Phosphorus[1] mmol	Magnesium mmol	Sodium mmol	Potassium mmol	Chloride[4] mmol	Iron µmol	Zinc µmol	Copper µmol	Selenium µmol	Iodine µmol
0–3 months	13.1	13.1	2.2	9	20	9	30	60	5	0.1	0.4
4–6 months	13.1	13.1	2.5	12	22	12	80	60	5	0.2	0.5
7–9 months	13.1	13.1	3.2	14	18	14	140	75	5	0.1	0.5
10–12 months	13.1	13.1	3.3	15	18	15	140	75	5	0.1	0.5
1–3 years	8.8	8.8	3.5	22	20	22	120	75	6	0.2	0.6
4–6 years	11.3	11.3	4.8	30	28	30	110	100	9	0.3	0.8
7–10 years	13.8	13.8	8.0	50	50	50	160	110	11	0.4	0.9
Males											
11–14 years	25.0	25.0	11.5	70	80	70	200	140	13	0.6	1.0
15–18 years	25.0	25.0	12.3	70	90	70	200	145	16	0.9	1.0
19–50 years	17.5	17.5	12.3	70	90	70	160	145	19	0.9	1.0
50+ years	17.5	17.5	12.3	70	90	70	160	145	19	0.9	1.0
Females											
11–14 years	20.0	10.0	11.5	70	80	70	260[5]	140	13	0.6	1.0
15–18 years	20.0	20.0	12.3	70	90	70	260[5]	110	16	0.8	1.1
19–50 years	17.5	17.5	10.9	70	90	70	260[5]	110	19	0.8	1.1
50+ years	17.5	17.5	10.9	70	90	70	160	110	19	0.8	1.1
Pregnancy	*	*	*	*	*	*	*	*	*	*	*
Lactation:											
0–4 months	+14.3	+14.3	+2.1	*	*	*	*	+90	+5	+0.2	*
4+ months	+14.3	+14.3	+2.1	*	*	*	*	+40	+5	+0.2	*

* No increment

[1] Phosphorus RNI is set equal to calcium in molar terms

[2] 1 mmol sodium = 23 mg

[3] 1 mmol potassium = 39 mg

[4] Corresponds to sodium 1 mmol = 35.5 mg

[5] Insufficient for women with high menstrual losses where the most practical way of meeting iron requirements is to take iron supplements

Table 30(b) Recommended daily amounts of some minerals for male and female population groups in the United Kingdom (*Dietary Reference Values for Food Energy and Nutrients for the United Kingdom*, HMSO Press; reproduced with the permission of the Controller of HMSO).

Age	Calcium mg	Phosphorus[1] mg	Magnesium mg	Sodium[2] mg	Potassium[3] mg	Chloride[4] mg	Iron mg	Zinc mg	Copper mg	Selenium μg	Iodine μg
0–3 months	525	400	55	210	800	320	1.7	4.0	0.2	10	50
4–6 months	525	400	60	280	850	400	4.3	4.0	0.3	13	60
7–9 months	525	400	75	320	700	500	7.8	5.0	0.3	10	60
10–12 months	525	400	80	350	700	500	7.8	5.0	0.3	10	60
1–3 years	350	270	85	500	800	800	6.9	5.0	0.4	15	70
4–6 years	450	350	120	700	1,100	1,100	6.1	6.5	0.6	20	100
7–10 years	550	450	200	1,200	2,000	1,800	8.7	7.0	0.7	30	110
Males											
11–14 years	1,000	775	280	1,600	3,100	2,500	11.3	9.0	0.8	45	130
15–18 years	1,000	775	300	1,600	3,500	2,500	11.3	9.5	1.0	70	140
19–50 years	700	550	300	1,600	3,500	2,500	8.7	9.5	1.2	75	140
50+ years	700	550	300	1,600	3,500	2,500	8.7	9.5	1.2	75	140
Females											
11–14 years	800	625	280	1,600	3,100	2,500	14.8[5]	9.0	0.8	45	130
15–18 years	800	625	300	1,600	3,500	2,500	14.8[5]	7.0	1.0	60	140
19–50 years	700	550	270	1,600	3,500	2,500	14.8[5]	7.0	1.2	60	140
50+ years	700	550	270	1,600	3,500	2,500	8.7	7.0	1.2	60	140
Pregnancy	*	*	*	*	*	*	*	*	*	*	*
Lactation:											
0–4 months	+550	+440	+50	*	*	*	*	+6.0	+0.3	+15	*
4+ months	+550	+440	+50	*	*	*	*	+2.5	+0.3	+15	*

* No increment

[1] Phosphorus RNI is set equal to calcium in molar terms

[2] 1 mmol sodium = 23 mg

[3] 1 mmol potassium = 39 mg

[4] Corresponds to sodium 1 mmol = 35.5 mg

[5] Insufficient for women with high menstrual losses where the most practical way of meeting iron requirements is to take iron supplements

Table 31   Safe daily intakes of some vitamins and minerals.

Nutrient	Safe intake
Vitamins:	
Pantothenic acid	
adults	3–7 mg
infants	1.7 mg
Biotin	10–200 µg
Vitamin E	
men	above 4 mg
women	above 3 mg
infants	0.4 mg/g polyunsaturated fatty acids
Vitamin K	
adults	1µg/kg
infants	10 µg
Minerals:	
Manganese	
adults	1.4 mg (26 µmol)
infants and children	16 µg (0.3 µmol)
Molybdenum	
adults	50–400 µg
infants, children and adolescents	0.5–1.5 µg/kg
Chromium	
adults	25 µg (0.5 µmol)
children and adolescents	0.1–1.0 µg (2–20 µmol)/kg
Fluoride (for infants only)	0.05 mg (3 µmol)/kg

How common are trace element deficiencies?

Except for iron and iodine, trace element deficiencies are relatively rare although zinc deficiency is becoming an increasingly recognized problem. Selenium deficiency has also been reported. Iron and iodine deficiencies lead to significant morbidity in the third world countries. In the more affluent countries including the UK, iron deficiency is common among the elderly and some Asian toddlers.

What are the functions of the trace elements and what are the symptoms of deficiency?

The trace metals are generally components of metallo–enzymes which ensure that the biochemical reactions in which they are involved proceed at rates compatible with health and life. Deficiency leads to a wide range of non-specific but often characteristic symptoms. Table 32 lists some of the biological functions of the trace elements and symptoms associated with their deficiency.

How safe are the essential trace elements at high doses?

Excessive intake of each of the trace elements is potentially toxic and potential toxic reactions are listed in Table 32.

Table 32 Some functions of essential trace elements and possible symptoms of deficiency.

Trace metal	Some biological functions	Some symptoms of deficiency	Potential toxicity
Chromium	Glucose metabolism	Glucose interolance	Undefined
Cobalt	Vitamin B_{12} activity Red blood cell formation	Unknown	Hearing problems, polycythaemia cardiomyopathy
Copper	Connective tissue metabolism, nerve function, haemopoiesis	Malabsorption, kwashiorkor, Wilson's disease (hepatotenticular degeneration)	Haematemesis, melaena
Iodine	Thyroid hormone synthesis	Cretinism, thyroid disorders	Hypothyroidism
Iron	Oxygen transport	Lethargy, dysphagia, breathlessness, anorexia	Gastrointestinal problems, liver and cardiovascular damage
Manganese	Synthesis of proteins and fatty acid metabolism	Weight loss, hypocholesterolaemia, prolongation of bleeding time	Parkinson-like symptoms
Molybdenum	Oxidase functions	Unknown	Gout-like symptoms
Selenium	Peroxidase activity antioxidant	Congestive cardiomyopathy	Hair loss, vomiting, finger nails abnormality
Zinc	Nucleic acid synthesis	Retarded growth hyperkeratosis Impaired immunity	Nausea, vomiting, colic

What are the main dietary sources of the trace elements?

Trace elements in foods often reflect the soil composition. In some parts of China, for example, the soil is selenium-deficient and symptoms of deficiency arise with the normal diet. However, some foods are known to be rich in certain minerals and Table 33 gives some examples.

Table 33   Sources of nutritionally important elements.

Mineral or trace element	Foods relatively rich in the element
Calcium	Dairy products
Chromium	Brewer's yeast, liver, fish
Cobalt	Meats, liver
Copper	Seafoods
Iodine	Seafoods
Iron	Red meats, cereals
Magnesium	Cereals, nuts, vegetables
Manganese	Vegetables, cereals
Molybdenum	Vegetables, cereals
Potassium	Fruits, fish, meats, nuts, cereals
Selenium	Seafoods, liver, whole grains
Zinc	Meats, seafoods, cereals

Who needs calcium supplements?

Most of the calcium in the body is in the bones and teeth. Only about 1% is found elsewhere in the body for metabolic and/or physiological, as opposed to structural, functions. The bone calcium is, however, in equilibrium with the calcium in blood and the metabolic role of calcium has priority over its structural function. Deficiency leads to rickets and osteoporosis.

Growing bones need calcium and milk is high in calcium. Therefore, children and adolescents and nursing mothers need increased calcium intakes. Dietary adjustment can meet most of the additional needs. Calcium supplements have recently been promoted for preventing post-menopausal osteoporosis but clinical trials have produced conflicting results and oestrogens are widely regarded as being the treatment of choice. However, since calcium supplements are generally safe and there are some data to support their use, dietary supplements should not be discouraged. It is possible that some highly active athletes may need additional calcium.

Are zinc supplements ever required?

Zinc supplements are used with success in *acrodermatitis enteropathica*, a rare hereditary disorder presenting with alopecia, diarrhoea and dermatitis. Hypogonadal dwarfism, as seen in some areas of Iran and Egypt, is also responsive to zinc supplements. Patients with impaired wound healing and low zinc levels may benefit from zinc supplements.

Are magnesium supplements useful?

Magnesium plays important roles in electrolyte homeostasis, particularly in the functioning of the sodium/potassium pump. Deficiency of magnesium leads to hyperexcitability of tissues and the cardiovascular consequences are the most worrying. Some patients on diuretics may be magnesium deficient and supplements have been suggested for such patients, particularly if they are concurrently receiving digoxin; however, this is not generally endorsed.

Precautions and when to refer

 Patients who complain of constant fatigue – serious underlying problems are possible.

 Avoid excessive doses of vitamins A and D.

 Excess intake of pyridoxine may lead to neurotoxicity.

Product options

Abidec Capsules
Abidec Drops
Adexolin Drops
Allbee with C Capsules
APS Vitamin Tablets
BC 500 Tablets
BC 500 with Iron Tablets
Becosym Forte Tablets
Becosym Syrup
Becosym Tablets
Bemax
Benadon Tablets
Benerva Compound
   Tablets
Benerva Tablets
Biovital Liquid
Biovital Tablets
Boots Vitamin & Iron Tonic
   Mixture

Calcium Factor 500
   Tablets
Calcium with Vitamin D
   Tablets BPC
Centurion Pastilles
Chewable Vitamin C
   Tablets
Complement Sustained
   Release Tablets
Concavit Capsules
Concavit Drops
Concavit Syrup
Cox Junior Multivitamin
   Chewable Tablets
Cox Multivitamin
   Chewable Tablets
Cox Multivitamin & Iron
   Chewable Tablets
Crookes One-A-Day
   Tablets

Crookes One-A-Day with
   Iron Tablets
Cytacon Liquid
Cytacon Tablets
Dalivit Drops
Dayovite Effervescent
   Granules
Efamol Plus Capsules
Ephynal Tablets
EPOC Capsules
Evans Multivitamin
   Capsules
Evans Multivitamin Plus
   Iron Capsules
Fesovit Spansule Sustained
   Release Capsules
Fesovit Z Spansule
   Capsules
Forceval Capsules
Forceval Junior Capsules

Formula AR-19 Tablets

Gaba with Inositol & Niacinamide Tablets

Galfer-Vit Capsules

Gammaoil Premium Capsules

Halaurant Liquid

Haliborange Chewable Tablets

Haliborange Multivitamin Plus Calcium and Iron Tablets

Halycitrol Syrup Emulsion

Iron 40 mg Tablets

Iron Jelloids Tablets

Ketovite Sugar Free Mixture

Ladycare No. 1 Tablets

Ladycare No. 2 Tablets

Ladycare No. 3 Tablets

Lance B+C Tablets

Lederplex Liquid

Maxi-Hair Hypo-Allergenic Formulation

Mega Mineral Complex Tablets

Minadex Syrup

Minamino CO Syrup

Multivitamin and Minerals with Ginseng Extract Capsules

Natures Best B-12 1000 MCG/Sorbitol Tablets

Natures Best Beta Carotene Plus CE & Selenium Tablets

Natures Best Bioflavonoids 500 mg Complex Tablets

Natures Best C-500 mg/ Rose Hips & Bioflavonoids Tablets

Natures Best Calcium 250 mg Tablets, C-Vit Tablets

Natures Best Calcium 500 mg Tablets

Natures Best Chlorophyll Thymol Tablets

Natures Best Choice 250 mg/Inositol Tablets

Natures Best Choline 500 mg Tablets

Natures Best Chromium 200 mcg Tablets

Natures Best Copper Tablets 3 mg

Natures Best DL-Methionine Tablets 500 mg

Natures Best Glucomannan Slim Plan Capsules

Natures Best Granular Lecithin Granules

Natures Best GTF Chromium Tablets 200 mcg

Natures Best Inositol 750 mg Tablets

Natures Best L-Arginine 500 mg Tablets

Natures Best L-Aspartic Acid 500 mg Tablets

Natures Best L-Cysteine 500 mg Tablets

Natures Best L-Glutathione 50 mg Tablets

Natures Best L-Histidine 500 mg Tablets

Natures Best L-Isoleucine 500 mg Tablets

Natures Best L-Leucine 500 mg Tablets

Natures Best L-Methionine 500 mg Tablets

Natures Best L-Ornithine 500 mg Capsules

Natures Best L-Threonine 400 mg Tablets

Natures Best L-Tyrosine 500 mg Tablets

Natures Best L-Valine 500 mg Tablets

Natures Best Magnesium 200 mg Tablets

Natures Best Manganese 50 mg Tablets

Natures Best Mineral Complex Amino Chelate Tablets

Natures Best Nicotinic Acid 500 mg Time-Release Tablets

Natures Best PABA 500 mg Tablets

Natures Best Pantothenic Acid 500 mg (Vitamin B-5) Tablets

Natures Best Potassium 99 mg Tablets

Natures Best RNA 100 mg 500 mg Tablets

Natures Best RNA 500 mg/DNA 100 mg Tablets

Natures Best Rutin 500 mg Tablets

Natures Best Selenium + A + C + E Tablets

Natures Best Selenium 1000 mcg Tablets

Natures Best Taurine 500 mg Tablets

Natures Best VItamin A Capsules

Natures Best Vitamin B-1 500 mg Tablets

Natures Best Vitamin B-2 500 mg Tablets

Natures Best Vitamin B-6 500 mg Tablets

Natures Best Vitamin E Cream

Naudicelle Capsules

Naudicelle Plus Capsules

Nova-C Chewable Tablets

Octovit Tablets

Orovite '7' Ganules

Orovite Syrup

Orovite Tablets

Paxadon Tablets

Pharmaton Tablets

Phillips Iron Tonic Tablets

Phylan/100-L-Phenylalanine 100 mg Tablets

Phyllosan Tablets

Pil Food Capsules

Plurivite Multivitamin Tablets

Redelan Tablets

Redoxon C Chewable Tablets

Redoxon Effervescent Tablets

Redoxon Tablets

Ribena Children's VItamins A C D Tablets

Sanatogen B6 Capsules

Sanatogen B Complex Tablets

Sanatogen Children's Vitamin Tablets

Sanatogen Cod Liver Oil Capsules 300 mg

Sanatogen Korean Ginseng Capsules

Sanatogen Multivitamin Plus Calcium Tablets

Sanatogen Multivitamin Plus Iron Tablets

Sanatogen Multivitamin Tablets

Sanatogen Omega 3 Capsules

Sanatogen Vit B CO Tablets

Sanatogen Vit C Tablets 30 mg

Sanatogen Vit C Tablets 500 mg

Sanatogen Vitamin E Capsules 400 iu

Scott's Emulsion

Sea-Cal Tablets

Selenium-ACE Tablets

Seven Seas Cholesterol-Free Lecithin Capsules

Seven Seas Cider + 3 Diet Aid Capsules

Seven Seas Cod Liver Oil

Seven Seas Cod Liver Oil Capsules

Seven Seas Maxepa Capsules

Seven Seas Multivitamin and Mineral Capsules

Seven Seas Orange Syrup

Seven Seas Orange Syrup and Cod Liver Oil

Seven Seas Super VItamin B6 Capsules

Seven Seas Super Vitamin E Capsules

Seven Seas Traditional & Cherry Cod Liver Oil Capsules

Seven Seas Vitamin B Complex Extra B6 & Brewers Yeast Capsules

Seven Seas Vitamin C-Plus Capsules

Seven Seas Wheat Germ Oil Capsules

Smokers Formula Tablets

Stress B Supplement Tablets

Sunnimax Tablets

Super Gammaoil Marine Capsules

Super Plenamins Tablets

Super Selenium Complex Tablets

Super Zinc-C Lozenges

Surbex T Tablets

Tandem IQ Tablets

Top C Tablets

Totavit Capsules

Vita-E Gels Capsules

Vita-E Gelucaps Chewable Tablets

Vita-E Succinate Tablets

Vitamin C Tablets BP

Vitaminised Iron Tonic Tablets with Yeast

Vitamin Capsules BPC

Vitaplus with Iron Tablets

Vitrite Syrup

Vitaplus Tablets

Vykmin Capsules

Zincold 23 Tablets

Warts

What are warts?

Warts are localized areas of hyperkeratinization induced by viruses of the papo-vavirus group. Several types are known and the most common affect the hands, feet and anogenital areas. The margin of the eye-lids are also commonly affected.

How serious are warts?

Warts are usually quite benign and resolve spontaneously with time. Their presence is not marked by any signs of systemic disturbance and pain is characteristically absent. Deep plantar warts may, however, become painful as a result of continued pressure on the hard masses which eventually damage surrounding tissues. Occasionally warts appear to spread rapidly with single lesions developing into clusters. The patient is alarmed and reassurance is then necessary.

How do warts develop?

Contact of the viral particles with the skin does not normally lead to warts. Infection appears to set in only in the presence of damaged or highly hydrated skin. Circumstantial evidence is provided by the distribution of the lesions on the body surface and by the apparent high level of cross-infection at swimming pools, sports centres and saunas.

How should warts be treated?

The isolated wart should be left alone but when faced with the persistent patient, a suitable topical application may be recommended. Salicylic acid has stood the test of time and is probably the agent of first choice. By weakening the cement material of the epidermal layers, shedding is stimulated and with it the wart. The keratolytic agent does not differentiate between healthy and infected keratin and protection of the surrounding area with soft paraffin is required. The use of wart plasters achieves both objectives, namely treatment and protection of surrounding healthy skin, simultaneously.

Formaldehyde and gluteraldehyde are also effective. Their mode of action is not well defined but they possess some antiviral activity and may exert some of their activity through a drying effect. Soaking in warm water for a few minutes prior to application of the topical medication may help penetration and enhance activity. Formaldehyde soaks are ideal for the treatment of a number of warts affecting the same area such as the soles. Warts in the anogenital area and on the face should be treated under medical supervision.

What advice should be given to patients in order to minimize spread of the infection?

Patients with plantar warts should avoid using swimming pools, saunas and so on without wearing special protective socks. Treatment can typically take weeks and the patient should therefore be warned.

Precautions and when to refer

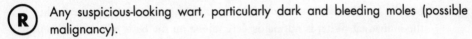 Any suspicious-looking wart, particularly dark and bleeding moles (possible malignancy).

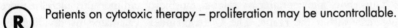 Patients on cytotoxic therapy – proliferation may be uncontrollable.

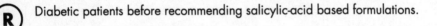 Diabetic patients before recommending salicylic-acid based formulations.

Product options

Salicylic acid containing products
Bazuka Gel (salicylic acid, lactic acid)
Compound W Liquid (salicylic acid)
Cuplex Gel (salicylic acid, lactic acid)
Duofilm Solution (salicylic acid, lactic acid)

Occlusal Application (salicylic acid)
Salactol Paint (salicylic acid, lactic acid)
Salatac Gel (salicylic acid, lactic acid)

Formaldehyde-containing product
Veracur Gel

Glutaraldehyde-containing products
Glutarol Solution   Verucasep Gel

Weight control

What is obesity?

Obesity is an increase in body weight beyond the acceptable range for the height of the individual. What is normal is determined on the basis of actuarial considerations. Thus above a given range of weights, morbidity and mortality increase more sharply than within the range. The Quetelet index, calculated by dividing the weight in kilograms by the height squared, in metres, provides a convenient measure of obesity. The normal range is between 20 to 25. Gross obesity is associated with Quetelet indices of 40 or higher while indices beyond 50 should cause serious concern.

How common is obesity?

A recent survey showed that about 5% of those surveyed at age 36 were at least 20% above the maximum of their normal weight ranges. There was marked variability in incidence of obesity between the sexes and social classes. Thus, 9.6% of the men in social class V were overweight while in class I, the corresponding figure was 4.2%. Among the women, the corresponding figures were 20.6 and 7.1 respectively. An equally recent survey shows that perhaps as many as 20% of all adults in the UK are above the desirable weight. The problem may be even worse in some other countries.

What causes obesity?

Obesity results from a calorie intake in excess of body requirements for the maintenance of normal body weight. However, obesity does not necessarily mean excessive food intake relative to other individuals since metabolic rates show wide inter-subject variability. Different subjects may also show different thermogenic responses to the intake of food. The slim may well be lucky because they burn off fat more readily than the obese.

Is it true that proteins are less likely to cause obesity?

This is not strictly true since weight for weight, proteins contain as many calories as carbohydrates (4 Kcal per gram) and excess food intake, whether the food is in the form of carbohydrates, fats or proteins, leads to laying down of fat in adipose cells below the skin or around internal organs. However fats (9 Kcal/gram) and alcohol (7cal/gram) contain more calories, weight for weight, than do proteins. Since satiety is largely controlled by the volume of food consumed, ingesting low calorie, high bulk foods may be helpful in reducing calorie intake.

What controls appetite?

Appetite is under both peripheral and central control. In the central nervous system, appetite regulation takes place mainly in the hypothalamus through a series of neurotransmitters. For a long time, nutrient control or appetostatic theories suggesting that glucose utilization or amino acid release regulated appetite, were widely accepted. One recent theory suggests that opiod peptides maintain a tonic drive to eat. This theory is supported by the observations that naloxone inhibits feeding. The kappa opiate receptors are thought to be particularly important in appetite control. Glucose levels modulate the effects of opiates on feeding behaviour thus providing some link between the early glucostatic theory and the opiate receptor theory of appetite control.

Neuropeptides such as calcitonin suppress appetite as does corticotropin-releasing factor (CRF). Increased CRF function is in fact thought to provide the pathophysiological basis for anorexia nervosa. Other neuropeptides including bombesin and thyrotropin-releasing hormone also appear to suppress feeding. Additionally, monoamines and in particular 5-hydroxytryptamine (serotonin) and dopamine are thought to modulate feeding behaviour. Satiety, for example, is thought to be under positive serotoninergic control and it is well known that the antihistaminic 5-hydroxytryptamine inhibitor, cyproheptadine, stimulates appetite while serotonin agonists induce anorexia. Dopamine blockade inhibits opiate-induced feeding.

Peripherally, bombesin, a gastric hormone, exerts a potent satiating effect. Cholecystokinin, released from the small intestines, inhibits feeding and somatostatin and pancreatic glucagon may be involved. There is also evidence to suggest that changes in glucose metabolism during feeding signal satiety.

Why is obesity undesirable?

Gross obesity is aesthetically and socially undesirable, although fashions change and at one time mild obesity was regarded as sexually attractive. In some societies, obesity is still desirable. Aside from aesthetic unacceptability in some circles, obesity is undesirable because of its health implications. It has, for example, been estimated that life expectancy is reduced by at least 1 year for each 10% increase in weight above the normal range. Disorders which have been specifically associated with obesity are hypertension, coronary heart disease, atherosclerosis and diabetes. Gallstones, gout, hiatus hernia and varicose veins are also more common among the obese than among normal weight individuals. Obesity may also put additional physical strain on patients suffering from chronic heart diseases, respiratory diseases and osteoarthritis.

How can weight reduction be achieved?

Weight reduction can only be achieved by reducing food intake so that there is a negative balance between calorie consumption and energy expenditure. The simplest method is by voluntary control of food intake but this is also the most difficult regimen to adhere to. Most obese individuals need recourse to anorectic agents in order to reduce food intake and low calorie foods may help. Effective anorectic agents include amphetamine and fenfluramine. Amphetamine is potentially addictive and is now rarely used for weight reduction. Fenfluramine is still widely used.

In some countries, phenylpropanolamine is available as a non-prescription anorectic agent but its use in immediate-release formulations has been associated with fatal hypertensive crises. Controlled-release formulations have not led to the same problem and an osmotic system (Acutrim) is widely used in the USA but so far not in the UK.

How long does it take to lose 10 pounds in weight?

A pound of fatty tissue is equivalent to about 3500 Kcal. Most sedentary women would have a daily energy requirement of about 2000 Kcal. On a very low calorie diet, such women would develop a deficit of about 1700 Kcal each day. This is the equivalent to about half a pound of fatty tissue. Men would lose about three quarters of a pound of fat each day. Therefore on average, most obese women would lose 10 pounds in about 3 weeks and it would be unrealistic to expect any more rapid weight loss. Moderate dieting involving a consumption of say 1500 Kcal per day would take about a week to lead to a loss of one pound in weight. Such moderate dieting needs more persistence and motivation than the very low calorie diets, as up to 3 months may be required for a loss of 10 pounds in weight.

What is the Cambridge Diet?

The Cambridge Diet is a very low calorie balanced diet providing a daily intake of 330 Kcals in the form of powder sachets for reconstitution in water. The primary sources of protein (33 g) are low-fat milk solids and soya flour. Fat (3 g) is provided by soya flour while carbohydrates (42 g) are included as lactose. Vitamins, minerals and trace elements are added at 100% of the UK and USA recommended allowances. Each daily intake contains 7 g of fibre. The diet was first developed by a nutritionist at the University of Cambridge and is now commercially exploited by a company.

Is the Cambridge Diet any better than the many previously-developed slimming diets?

Over the years, a variety of slimming diets have been put forward and very low calorie diets (VLCDs) received particular prominence a few years ago because of a number of deaths associated with their use. The VLCDs provide less than 600 Kcal daily for up to several weeks and therefore the Cambridge Diet is an example of a VLCD. However, the Cambridge Diet has a high quality amino acid profile, unlike the early VLCDs which were deficient in several essential amino acids. The Cambridge Diet is also formulated as a full formula product with added micro-nutrients, minerals and trace elements. Most early VLCDs were intended to be used with additional supplements but not all patients took them as recommended. The widespread use of the Cambridge Diet has so far not led to reports of serious adverse reactions which characterized the use of the early VLCDs. Based on current evidence the Cambridge Diet would therefore appear to be safer than the early VLCDs.

Should one then assume that the Cambridge Diet is totally safe?

This should not be assumed. Use of any VLCD, including the Cambridge Diet, should be avoided by insulin-dependent diabetics, patients with recent cardio-vascular problems, pregnant and lactating women and children. There is also insufficient experience of the long-term use and of the on-off use of the Cambridge Diet.

Are digestion inhibitors useful in dieting?

This is an attractive approach to weight control since inhibition of digestion should theoretically lead to reduced calorie absorption and hence weight loss. The so-called 'starch blockers', containing starch amylase inhibitors, extracted from the red kidney bean (*Phaseolus vulgaris*), are promoted as one such slimming aid but clinical evaluation has shown them to be ineffective. Flatulence and gastro-intestinal disturbance are common problems associated with the use of starch blockers.

Is it true that non-absorbable fats will soon be available as calorie-free fats?

Sucrose polyester is currently being investigated as a calorie-free fat substitute. The polyester is made up of a sucrose molecule with as many as eight molecules of fatty acids linked by enzyme-resistant covalent bonds. The polyester, which is therefore non-absorbable and calorie-free, is already on sale in Japan as a food stabilizer rather than as a fat substitute. The Food and Drug Administration of the USA has recently approved the use of sucrose polyester and generated much controversy in the process.

Spirulina has recently been promoted as a slimming aid. What is it and is it useful for slimming?

Spirulina are filamentous cyanobacteria characterized by spiral-shaped chains of cells enclosed in a thin sheath. Spirulina are also referred to as a blue green algae and form a genus of the Oscillatoriaceae family. The species *S. platensis* forms large floating mats on lakes in certain parts of Chad. The mats are sun-dried and have been used as a food item by some Chadians for a long time. A different species, *S. maxima* apparently grew well in Mexican lakes and was used as a food by the Aztecs. With this historical background, some manufacturers did not find it too hard to persuade many consumers that spirulina were the ultimate health food. A large proportion of the spirulina currently marketed is of cultivated variety.

Spirulina are certainly rich in protein, which makes up 70% of their dry weight. The amino acid composition appears to be very good but not as well balanced as egg albumin or casein. They are also rich in the essential fatty acids linoleic acid and gamma linolenic acid. However, the claimed magical properties of spirulina remain elusive. They are only likely to be useful as a slimming aid when consumed as part of a calorie-controlled diet. With a price tag which makes this protein as expensive gram for gram as caviar, calorie control may not be too difficult if it is used as the only food source.

Are diabetic foods useful as slimming aids?

Low calorie diabetic foods are clearly suitable as slimming aids. However, diabetic foods based on calorigenic ingredients such as sorbitol and lycasin would not be. Foods sweetened solely by saccharin, aspartame and acesulfame would be appropriate if the other components were low-calorie items.

Precautions and when to refer

 When obesity is severe enough to cause other health problems.

 Phenylpropanolamine-based products should not be recommended for weight control. At effective doses adverse effects may be serious.

Index